FREE Study Skills DVD Offer

Dear Customer,

Thank you for your purchase from Mometrix! We consider it an honor and privilege that you have purchased our product and want to ensure your satisfaction.

As a way of showing our appreciation and to help us better serve you, we have developed a Study Skills DVD that we would like to give you for <u>FREE</u>. **This DVD covers our "best practices" for studying for your exam, from using our study materials to preparing for the day of the test.**

All that we ask is that you email us your feedback that would describe your experience so far with our product. Good, bad or indifferent, we want to know what you think!

To get your **FREE Study Skills DVD**, email <u>freedvd@mometrix.com</u> with "FREE STUDY SKILLS DVD" in the subject line and the following information in the body of the email:

   a. The name of the product you purchased.

   b. Your product rating on a scale of 1-5, with 5 being the highest rating.

   c. Your feedback. It can be long, short, or anything in-between, just your impressions and experience so far with our product. Good feedback might include how our study material met your needs and will highlight features of the product that you found helpful.

   d. Your full name and shipping address where you would like us to send your free DVD.

If you have any questions or concerns, please don't hesitate to contact me directly.

Thanks again!

Sincerely,

Jay Willis
Vice President
<u>jay.willis@mometrix.com</u>
1-800-673-8175

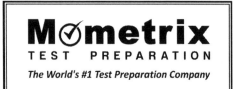

Informatics Nurse Exam
SECRETS

Study Guide
Your Key to Exam Success

Informatics Test Review for the
Informatics Nurse Exam

Published by
Mometrix Test Preparation
Informatics Nurse Exam Secrets Test Prep Team

Written and edited by the Informatics Nurse Exam Secrets Test Prep Staff

Printed in the United States of America

This paper meets the requirements of ANSI/NISO Z39.48-1992 (Permanence of Paper).

Mometrix offers volume discount pricing to institutions. For more information or a price quote, please contact our sales department at sales@mometrix.com or 888-248-1219.

Mometrix Test Preparation is not affiliated with or endorsed by any official testing organization. All organizational and test names are trademarks of their respective owners.

ISBN 13: 978-1-60971-976-0
ISBN 10: 1-60971-976-X

Dear Future Exam Success Story:

Congratulations on your purchase of our study guide. Our goal in writing our study guide was to cover the content on the test, as well as provide insight into typical test taking mistakes and how to overcome them.

Standardized tests are a key component of being successful, which only increases the importance of doing well in the high-pressure high-stakes environment of test day. How well you do on this test will have a significant impact on your future, and we have the research and practical advice to help you execute on test day.

The product you're reading now is designed to exploit weaknesses in the test itself, and help you avoid the most common errors test takers frequently make.

How to use this study guide

We don't want to waste your time. Our study guide is fast-paced and fluff-free. We suggest going through it a number of times, as repetition is an important part of learning new information and concepts.

First, read through the study guide completely to get a feel for the content and organization. Read the general success strategies first, and then proceed to the content sections. Each tip has been carefully selected for its effectiveness.

Second, read through the study guide again, and take notes in the margins and highlight those sections where you may have a particular weakness.

Finally, bring the manual with you on test day and study it before the exam begins.

Your success is our success

We would be delighted to hear about your success. Send us an email and tell us your story. Thanks for your business and we wish you continued success.

Sincerely,

Mometrix Test Preparation Team

Need more help? Check out our flashcards at: http://MometrixFlashcards.com/InfoNurse

TABLE OF CONTENTS

Top 20 Test Taking Tips

1. Carefully follow all the test registration procedures
2. Know the test directions, duration, topics, question types, how many questions
3. Setup a flexible study schedule at least 3-4 weeks before test day
4. Study during the time of day you are most alert, relaxed, and stress free
5. Maximize your learning style; visual learner use visual study aids, auditory learner use auditory study aids
6. Focus on your weakest knowledge base
7. Find a study partner to review with and help clarify questions
8. Practice, practice, practice
9. Get a good night's sleep; don't try to cram the night before the test
10. Eat a well balanced meal
11. Know the exact physical location of the testing site; drive the route to the site prior to test day
12. Bring a set of ear plugs; the testing center could be noisy
13. Wear comfortable, loose fitting, layered clothing to the testing center; prepare for it to be either cold or hot during the test
14. Bring at least 2 current forms of ID to the testing center
15. Arrive to the test early; be prepared to wait and be patient
16. Eliminate the obviously wrong answer choices, then guess the first remaining choice
17. Pace yourself; don't rush, but keep working and move on if you get stuck
18. Maintain a positive attitude even if the test is going poorly
19. Keep your first answer unless you are positive it is wrong
20. Check your work, don't make a careless mistake

Foundations of Practice

Professional Practice

Roles Played by the Informatics Nurse

The following are some of the **roles** that the informatics nurse must play:
- **Developing informatics theories:** Assemble what sort of information should be captured on the system and how the data should be analyzed.
- **Analyzing the information needs of the organization:** Sort through the large amounts of data collected to determine the best information for the organization.
- **Helping the organization choose computer systems:** Assist in the system requirements, both for now and in the near future.
- **Customizing purchased computer systems:** Work with IT to customize the system so that it will be the most useful.
- **Designing computer information systems:** Assist IT in the overall design of the system.
- **Testing new or upgraded computer systems:** Conduct robust tests of the system when changes or upgrades are performed.
- **Teaching other people to use the computer system:** Set up training and education programs to encourage the most effective use of the system.

Informatics Nurse Responsibilities

The following is a list of **responsibilities** that are required of the informatics nurse:
- Teaching the policies involved with information systems.
  - This includes the standard operating procedures and system security features.
- Deciding the effectiveness of the computer system.
  - This is based on overall performance (e.g., system response time) and how well the system design is working.
- Making sure the system works as it was designed to.
  - By verifying that the system produces results that are expected and troubleshooting problems.
- Deciding when computer systems need to be upgraded.
  - This is based on gauging the obsolescence of the hardware and system compatibility with modern software.
- Finding new ways to use technology in nursing.
  - By looking for new and novel applications of technology.
- Ensuring compliance in regulations regarding patient information.
  - This includes the patient privacy regulations.
- Managing projects as needed.
- Conducting research into the field of nursing informatics.

Differences Between Clinical Nurses and Those Nurses Who Specialize in Informatics

The focus of a traditional **clinical nurse** revolves around taking care of patients. Their use of computerized systems is limited to the user level (i.e., enough knowledge to operate the equipment and enter data). Their concentration is on the accuracy of the information that they are interpreting or giving to other caregivers. They are trained to handle malfunctions and are used as a feedback source for the informatics developers. Their opinion of the computerized systems is key as to whether or not the system is successful.

Nurses who **specialize in informatics** focus on the information systems. They worry about the security and stability of the systems installed at their facility. They are also very adept at troubleshooting problems (especially at the user level). They make sure the systems are as user friendly as possible and, more importantly, reduce the number of tasks the traditional clinical nurse has to perform in their routine day. Efficiency and enhanced productivity are the key goals of the informatics nurse.

Essential Elements in the Practice of Nursing Informatics

The essential **elements** within the practice of **nursing informatics** include traditional nursing aspects such as:
- Focus on the patient and their well-being.
- Healthcare in general. Keeping up to date on the latest state of the art in terms of nursing.
- Working environment. This includes how things are laid out (to avoid errors and make things as efficient as possible).
- Working with others. How to interact effectively with other healthcare practitioners and coworkers.

In terms of informatics, the related skills include:
- Knowledge of data structures (including metastructures).
- Knowledge of computer networking.
- Knowledge of computer hardware.
- Information system training skills.

Formal education includes:
- A minimum of bachelor's degree in nursing or another relevant field
- Continuing education in informatics nursing, such as working toward a graduate degree

Framework for Nursing Informatics

The **American Nurses Association** (ANA) has laid out **standards** for the informatics nurse specialist. These standards are based on a "problem-solving framework," which includes both traditional aspects of nursing as well as those aspects more specific to the informatics nurse. The standards are:
- Assessment
- Problem or Issues
- Outcomes Identification
- Planning
- Implementation
    - Coordination of Activities
    - Health Teaching, Health Promotion and Education for Informatics Solutions
    - Consultation
- Evaluation
- Education
- Professional Practice Evaluation

- Quality of Practice
- Collegiality
- Collaboration
- Ethics
- Research
- Resource Utilization
- Advocacy
- Leadership

The ANA has also set standards for the performance that informatics nurses should attain. The performance issues include quality assurance, review of performance evaluation methods, and ensuring that the practice of nursing informatics is effective. The informatics nurse should also work to create guidelines for research, ethics, peer cooperation, allocation of resources, and effective communication. Finally, they should be willing to help other nurses who want to improve their skills in informatics and computer science.

Definition, Scope, and Functional Areas of the Informatics Nurse Specialist

The informatics nurse is one who works in informatics because of experience or interest in the field but has not received formal training; an **informatics nurse specialist (INS)** has completed graduate studies in informatics and may also have certification. According to the **American Nurses Association**, nursing informatics is a nursing specialty integrating nursing, computer sciences, and information sciences, which support professionals and patients in decision-making through information processes and technology. INS functions include:
- Providing tools for standardized documentation.
- Managing information and analyzing data.
- Re-engineering information processes and promoting standardization.
- Participating in research and collection of data.
- Providing nursing management and administration.
- Serving as a consultant in the field of informatics.
- Promoting and providing professional development activities, including training of human–computer interaction systems.
- Advocating for changes in policies.
- Serving as advocate for staff and patients.
- Ensuring implementation of electronic health records and computerized physician order entry systems.
- Providing support to clinical applications.

Implications of Health Care Reform

Health care reform initiatives are spurring the switch from paper to electronic health records and sharing of health care information among health care providers, increasing the demand for health information technology and people with expertise in informatics. New programs have been developed to focus on wellness with an increased emphasis on cost-effective measures because of increases in health costs. Internal data analysis and research are becoming important means by which to identify waste, institute best practices, and reduce costs. Increasing numbers of people are covered by health plans, even those with preexisting conditions, placing more demand on health care providers for services. There is an increased need for health literacy so that people are better informed about the services available, especially those newly insured. Medicaid costs have increased, resulting in some cutbacks in care. Early transfer from acute care facilities to extended care or home health care is also increasing.

American Nursing Informatics Association (ANIA) and Alliance for Nursing Informatics (ANI)

American Nursing Informatics Association (ANIA): ANIA is an organization that merged 2 existing informatics organization and aims to provide an organization for nurses and others interested in nursing informatics and to advance the profession. There are 4 ANIA regions: West, central, northeast and southeast. ANIA provides an interactive website and resources for members, an online digital library, webinars, continuing education courses, an open forum, a monthly electronic newsletter, and an annual ANIA conference.

Alliance for Nursing Informatics (ANI): ANI is a collaboration of different nursing informatics groups and includes organizations representing different types of nursing, such as AORN and ASPAN, as well as individual members and groups involved in the field of informatics. ANI serves as an intermediary to promote communication, education, and professional development. Members receive an online subscription to *Computer Information Nursing* (CIN) as well as news updates.

Evidence-Based Practice

Evidence-based practice is the use of current research and individual values in practice to establish a plan of care for each individual. Research may be the result of large studies of best practices or individual research from observations in practice about the effectiveness of treatment. Evidence-based practice requires a commitment to ongoing research and outcomes evaluations. Many resources are available, such as the *Guide to Clinical Preventive Services* by the Agency for Healthcare Research and Quality of the U. S. Department of Health and Human Services (http://www.ahrq.gov/clinic/cps3dix.htm). Evidence-based practice requires a thorough understanding of research methods to evaluate the results and determine if they can be generalized. Results must also be evaluated in terms of cost-effectiveness. Steps to evidence-based practice include:
- Making a diagnosis.
- Researching and analyzing results.
- Applying research findings to a plan of care.
- Evaluating outcomes.

Developing Guidelines Based on Evidence

Steps to **developing evidence-based practice guidelines** include the following:
- **Focus on the topic/methodology:** This includes outlining possible interventions/treatments for review, choosing individual populations and settings, and determining significant outcomes. Search boundaries (e.g., journals, studies, dates of studies) should be determined.
- **Evidence review:** This includes review of literature, critical analysis of studies, and a summary of results, including pooled meta-analysis.
- **Expert judgment:** Recommendations based on personal experience from a number of experts may be used, especially if there is inadequate evidence based on review, but this subjective evidence should be explicitly acknowledged.
- **Policy considerations:** This includes cost-effectiveness, access to care, insurance coverage, availability of qualified staff, and legal implications.

- **Policy:** A written policy must be completed with recommendations. Common practice is to use letter guidelines, with "A" the most highly recommended, usually based on the quality of supporting evidence.
- **Review:** The completed policy should be submitted to peers for review and comments before instituting the policy.

Integrating Evidence-Based Practice

Evidence-based practice must be part of the mission and goal of a health care organization, and **strategies** to attain this must be supported at all levels. Information technology tools, such as internet capability or access to information databases, should be available at the point of care so that health care providers are able to access journal articles and other clinical information. Links may be available through the patient's health risk evaluation as well. All staff should receive training in the use of equipment and methods of researching and retrieving information and have an understanding of how to interpret research findings; the inability of health care providers to understand and interpret findings can be a significant barrier to evidence-based practice. Because evidence-based practice often results in change, institutional support for change must be evident and may involve incentives. Continuing education classes should be available on-site to help health care providers gain the research skills they need.

Model of Integration

Integrating the results of data analysis and research into performance improvement or best practice guidelines varies from one organization to another, depending on the **model of integration** that the organization uses:
- **Organizational:** Processes for improvement are identified, and teams or individuals are selected to participate in different areas or departments, reporting to one individual, who monitors progress.
- **Functional/coordinated:** While staff specialties, such as risk management and quality management, are not integrated, they draw from the same data resources to determine issues related to quality of care and efficiency.
- **Functional/integrated:** While staff specialties remain, there is cross-training among specialties. A case management approach to individual care is used so that one person follows the progress of a patient through the system and coordinates with the various specialties, such as infection control and quality management.

Assuring Accuracy of Information

The following information attributes are important in assuring accuracy:
- **Objective reporting** - Information should be completely free from bias and reported accurately.
- **Comprehensive** - All the necessary information is available to complete reports and requests.
- **Appropriateness** - All users are able to access the information necessary to do their jobs.
- **Unambiguous** – The data is clearly defined in order to reduce errors.
- **Reliability** – When identical information is keyed in by different people, it should always be uniform in the system.
- **Up to Date** – The most recent information should be listed first.
- **Convenience** - It should not be difficult for users to locate the information they need.

Factors Necessary for Information Quality

Quality information is defined by the following factors:
- **Timeliness:** The necessary data is available (and retrievable) as needed.
- **Precision:** System dictionaries shall describe uniform wording and clear definitions.
- **Accuracy:** The data should be as error-free as possible.
- **Measurability:** The information should be quantifiable so that comparisons can be made.
- **Independently verifiable:** The integrity of the information remains constant regardless of the individual reporting it.
- **Availability:** The information should be accessible where it is needed. In the hospital or clinic environment, the information should usually be available at the patient's location.

Continuing Education Options

ANCC nurse informatics certification is granted for a 5-year period. Renewal requires 75 mandatory hours of **continuing education** and proof of activity in one to eight of the renewal categories, which include CE hours, academic credits (5 semester credits or 6 quarter credits, presentations (≥5 hours), publication or research, preceptor hours (120), professional service (≥2 years of volunteer service), practice hours (≥1000 hours), and retaking the assessment exam. Continuing education requirements include:
- At least half must be directly related to nurse informatics.
- At least half must be formally approved and provided by accredited provider and may include continuing nursing education (CNE) and continuing medical education (CME).
- Approved independent study or electronic learning may account for 100% of hours.
- Academic courses can be converted to contact hours: 1 semester credit equals 15 contact hours and 1 quarter credit equals 12.5 credit hours.

The nurse should maintain all records of completion of continuing education contact hours for 5 years, including the completion certificate that has the dates, title, provider, and number of contact hours.

Methodologies and Theories

Electronic Medical Records and Electronic Health Records

Although many in healthcare use the terms **electronic medical record (EMR)** and **electronic health record (EHR)** interchangeably, there are major distinctions between the two. The electronic medical record is created by a hospital or other health care delivery organization (CDO). The CDO owns the information in the EMR. The EMR consists of clinical documentation, orders, medications, treatments, and other clinical decision support, and is a legal record. The EHR includes information from EMRs, likely from multiple health care delivery organizations. The EHR relies on the information from the EMR to complete it. The EHR is owned by the patient and stakeholders, which could include the government, insurance companies, and healthcare providers among others. Important to the EMR is using controlled medical vocabulary so that information will be comparable among providers and other interested stakeholders. Currently in the United States the use of EHRs is limited, mostly due to many healthcare delivery organizations not having an established EMR using decided predetermined standards. There may soon be an increase in the number of organizations using EMRs with standardized language conducive to EHRs, as organizations now receive financial incentives to install EMR and EHR systems from health care reform.

Computer Science

Computer science is often misunderstood to be solely the study of computers. Computer science began long before modern computers were ever created. Computer science is the study of how information is manipulated to solve problems or answer questions. In essence, computational science has been automated by the technology of modern computers. There are many subfields within computer science including computer graphics, computational complexity theory, programming language theory, computer programming, and human/computer interaction or interface. The history of computer science is founded in mathematics and the two fields continue to influence one another. The first modern computers were designed to perform complex mathematical calculations related to projectile trajectories for the battlefield. Computer science may be thought of as the study of computation and its associated principles. More commonly, however, the education that computer scientists often receive focuses more on programming and the specific computational problems found in association with software engineering.

Management Science

Management science is the study of business decision-making using various analytical methods. There are several elements used in management science to help organizations make practical decisions:
- Strategic planning: Strategic planning is based on an organization's goals and mission.
- Morphological analysis: Morphological analysis looks at many different possible solutions in an attempt to come up with the most appropriate one.
- Influence diagrams: Influence diagrams use mathematical representations and graphs to solve problems.
- Problem structuring: A method used in management science is problem structuring, sometimes known as "soft-operations research."

Management science may also be called operations research. Some experts consider operations research primarily academic in nature (focusing only on making operations more productive and efficient) while management science is regarded to be more related to the process of making business decisions that effect more than operations.

DIKW Pyramid

The **DIKW pyramid** is a hierarchical method to show the relationship between the different elements of information processing and focuses on both function and structure. The lower levels contribute to the upper, and one can review a process by going up or down the pyramid:
- **Data** (base): Signs and signals, such as numbers, symbols, letters, and words used to describe empirical information that can be verified as factual although some models include subjective data, which cannot always be verified.
- **Information:** Results after context is applied to data that is entered into a system. Information can be inferred from data and used to answer questions.
- **Knowledge:** Knowledge considers information is terms of meaning, including subjective assessment. Knowledge derives from experience and facilitates development of theories and frameworks.
- **Wisdom** (apex): Wisdom is an appreciation and understanding of the whole and ethical considerations. Lower levels of the pyramid contribute to knowledge and wisdom, which form a frame of reference.

Fair Distribution of Health Information Access

The **fair distribution of health information access** relates to information specific to the individual (e.g., electronic health records), data (both aggregate and comparative), and knowledge-based information (e.g., journals, websites). While people should have access to health information, considerations must include the right to privacy, regulations regarding intellectual property, and equitable access to information. One problem with access is that many people are unaware of their rights or lack the training or tools to access information, so an important element of fair distribution must include providing public means of access, such as in libraries and through public health agencies and education (e.g., posters, handouts, videos) to educate the general public. People in rural or isolated areas may lack access to basic care and health information but may be served by telehealth services, using telecommunications to provide information and internet health resources.

Science of Unitary Human Beings

Martha E. Rogers developed the **science of unitary human beings** in the 1980s and 1990s. The individual is viewed as a unitary energy source within the larger universe, constantly interacting with the environment. The four primary characteristics of this theory include the following:
- **Energy field:** This is basic to all living and nonliving things.
- **Openness:** The individual and the environment exist together with an openness that allows a continuous exchange of energy.
- **Pattern:** This energy wave distinguishes and identifies the source of energy.
- **Pan-dimensionality:** This domain is nonlinear and not constrained by time or space, which are arbitrary means that people use to describe events.

Basic concepts derived from the above characteristics include the following:

- **Unitary human being:** Humans are energy fields that can be identified by patterns and characteristics. The holistic human cannot be predicted by parts but only by being viewed as a unified whole.
- **Environment:** The environmental energy field is integral to that of the human energy field.
- **Homeodynamics:** Good health and illness constitute part of the same continuum.

Interpersonal Relations Model of Nursing

Hildegard Peplau developed the **interpersonal relations model of nursing** in 1952, focusing on the quality of the nurse–client interaction. Peplau believed that patients deserved humane care by educated nurses and that they should be treated with dignity and respect. She also believed that the environment (i.e., social, psychosocial, physical) could affect health in a positive or negative manner. Peplau viewed the nurse as a person who could make a substantial difference for the patient and who acts as a "maturing force." The nurse can focus on the way in which patients react to their illness and can help patients to use illness as an opportunity for learning and maturing through the nurse–client interactions. The nurse helps the patient to understand the nature of his or her problem and to find solutions. Peplau's theory stresses the importance of collaboration between the patient and the nurse. The nurse–client relationship is viewed as a number of overlapping phases: orientation, identification of the problem, explanation of potential solutions, and resolution of the problem.

General Theory of Nursing

Dorothea Orem developed a **general theory of nursing** in 1959. Orem believed that the goal of nursing was to serve patients and assist them to provide self-care through three steps: identifying the reason a patient needs care, planning for delivery of care, and managing care. Orem's theory is actually a collection of three theories:

- **Self-care:** There are two agents, the self-care agent (i.e., the individual) and the dependent-care agent (i.e., the other caregiver). There are three categories of needs, consisting of universal needs (i.e., food, air), developmental needs (i.e., maturation or events), and health needs (i.e., illness, injury).
- **Self-care deficit:** This occurs if the self-care agent cannot provide for his or her own care. Nursing assists through five means: providing care, guiding, instructing, and adjusting the environment to help the patient in self-care.
- **Nursing systems:** Actions to meet the patient's self-care needs may be completely compensatory (i.e., patient is dependent), partly compensatory (i.e., patient provides some self-care), or supportive (i.e., patient needs assistance to provide self-care).

Total-Person Systems Model

Betty Neuman developed the **total-person systems model** of nursing in 1972. The concentric circle of variables (e.g., physiological, psychological, sociocultural, spiritual, developmental) provides defenses for the individual; these defenses should be considered simultaneously for the individual, who directly interacts with and is influenced by the environment. This model focuses on how the individual reacts to stress, using defense mechanisms and resistance, and how this feedback affects the individual's stability. Stressors are environmental forces that may provide negative or positive reactions, affecting the individual's stability. Stressors may be intrapersonal, interpersonal, or extrapersonal. The nurse intervenes to help the individual maintain stability and prevent negative effects. Interventions include the following:

- **Primary (health promotion, education):** Preventive steps are taken before a reaction to a stressor develops.
- **Secondary:** The goal is to prevent damage of the central core by facilitating internal resistance and by removal of stressors.
- **Tertiary:** Efforts are made to promote reconstitution and reduce energy needs, supporting the client after secondary interventions.

Founder of Modern Nursing

Florence Nightingale (1820–1910), **founder of modern nursing**, created one of the first training schools for nurses. Nightingale observed that the disciplined care provided to the sick by nuns was superior to the haphazard and untrained care of nurses in England. Based on her experiences in the Crimean War, Nightingale set standards for patient care that included sanitary conditions (e.g., cleanliness, improved ventilation, less crowding), adequate nutrition, and kindness. She used statistical analysis to show the number of deaths related to poor sanitation. Nightingale reformed the ways in which hospitals provided care for patients. She set standards for nursing and developed the Nightingale pledge, which is still recited by nurses at graduation ceremonies. Reciting this pledge, nurses swear that they will practice the profession faithfully, do no harm, maintain and elevate the standards of the nursing profession, maintain confidence in personal matters, aid the physician, and devote themselves to the welfare of the patient.

Nursing Process Theory

Ida Jean Orlando developed the **nursing process theory** in the late1950s and published them in 1961 in *The Dynamic Nurse–Patient Relationship,* based on her observations of what comprises good or bad nursing care. She theorized that the nursing process includes the following:

- **Behavior of the patient:** Behavior is an indication of need, which may be expressed directly or through actions.
- **Nurse's reaction:** The nurse must evaluate the needs of the patient based on perception and evaluation of this perception, exploring with the patient the meaning of the patient's behavior.
- **Subsequent nursing actions:** Actions are based on the nurse's determination of the patient's real needs, which may be different from expressed needs, and then finding the appropriate action to meet these needs. When the patient's needs are met, the patient's distress is decreased and his or her sense of well-being is improved.

Crisis Theory

Lee Ann Hoff developed the **crisis theory** of nursing. Crisis theory considers those stress-related events that are turning points in a person's life and can lead to danger or to opportunity. These may be health issues (e.g., cancer), environmental issues (e.g., an earthquake), criminal issues (e.g., rape), or any other issues that precipitate a crisis reaction. During a crisis, people are overwhelmed with anxiety and are unable to function effectively. Crisis management helps the person and those in his or her social network to deal with the crisis issues and reach resolution. The nurse and others, such as police, social workers, physicians, and ministers, depending on the type of crisis, are in the position to provide crisis intervention. Crisis care comprises a number of steps, including assessing the situation, making plans to resolve the crisis, implementing actions, and following up to ensure that the crisis has been resolved.

Information Theory

Claude Shannon devised the **information theory** in 1948, which is used to determine the effectiveness of communication systems, especially related to compressing, transmitting, and storing data. Shannon identified problems that required solutions. The essential factors in a system of communication include the source of power, the bandwidth, the noise, and the decoder/receiver. Information is carried by symbols, such as words or codes. The three steps involved in communication include encoding a message (e.g., bits, words, icons), transmission through a channel of communication (e.g., voice, radio, computer), and decoding when reaching a destination. Note that signal-to-noise indicates the ratio between a signal's magnitude and interfering "noise" magnitude. Another element is channel capacity, which determines the amount of information that can be transmitted with the smallest rate of error. Entropy refers to the amount of energy, code, or bits, required to communicate or store one symbol in the communication process. The lower the entropy, the more efficient the process of communication.

Transcultural Theory of Nursing

Madeline Leininger developed the **transcultural theory of nursing** in 1974, based on anthropological concepts. Transcultural nursing considers cultural issues as central to providing care and promotes study of cultural differences as they pertain to people's beliefs about illness, behavioral patterns, and caring behavior as well as nursing behavior. Leininger recognized that response to illness is often rooted in cultural beliefs and traditions. Based on research, the goal is to identify and provide care that is both culture-specific (i.e., fitting the needs of a specific cultural group based on their belief systems and behavior) and universal (i.e., based on belief systems and behavior that hold true for all cultures). Nurses are expected to determine the most appropriate approach to care, considering not only the needs of ethnic or minority populations but also gender issues. Transcultural theory tries to find ways to accommodate traditional belief systems with modern medicine and to prevent cultural conflict.

Philosophy of Human Caring

Jean Watson developed the **philosophy of human caring** in 1979. Watson focused on transpersonal caring, which views the individual holistically from the perspective of the interrelationship among health, sickness, and behavior with a nursing goal to promote health and prevent illness. Watson's theory encompasses ten caritas (methods of caring) the nurse can employ during opportunities to provide care and caring moments. The ten caritas include:
- Having loving kindness and equanimity.
- Being present and sustaining the spiritual beliefs of patient and self.
- Cultivating personal spiritual practice.
- Developing and maintaining a caring relationship.
- Supporting both negative and positive feelings of the patient.
- Being creative in caring.
- Providing teaching–learning experiences within the patient's frame of reference.
- Creating a physical and spiritual healing environment.
- Providing for basic human needs.
- Being open to spiritual concepts related to life and death of self and the patient.

Stages of Clinical Competence

Patricia Benner developed the **stages of clinical competence** for nurses based on the Dreyfus Model of Skill Acquisition in 1984. There are five stages of clinical competence for nurses:
- **Novice:** The novice has little experience, depends on rules and learned behavior, and is not able to adapt easily.
- **Advanced beginner:** The advanced beginner has some experience in coping with new situations and is able to formulate some principles of action.
- **Competent:** The competent nurse has 2–3 years of experience, has some mastery of new situations and goals, and can cope well but may require time for planning and lack flexibility.
- **Proficient:** The proficient nurse looks at situations holistically, relies on experience to determine goals and plans, can adapt plans to changing needs, and can make decisions based on the understanding of maxims.
- **Expert:** The expert nurse has a wealth of experience from which to draw and can provide care intuitively rather than relying on rules and maxims. The nurse is able to understand needs and determine quickly the most effective focus for providing care.

Theory of Cognitive Development

Jean Piaget's theory of cognitive development discusses how children assimilate new experiences and deal with them through accommodation. Piaget believed children go through stages of development, beginning with sensorimotor, which has six substages.

Stage	Age	Description
I	0–1 month of age	Reflexes (sucking, rooting, grasping, crying) are primary.
II	1–4 months of age	Reflexive behavior is replaced by voluntary behavior, recognizing a stimulus and a response (primary circular reactions).
III	4–8 months of age	There is an intensification of stage II, with children developing a sense of causality, time, and personal separateness. They begin to imitate and show different affects. They develop a sense of object permanence between 6 and 8 months (secondary circular reactions).
IV	9–12 months of age	This is a transitional stage with further intellectual development, including understanding that a hidden object is not gone. Children begin to behave with intention, to associate words and symbols (bye-bye) with events, and attempt to climb over obstacles.
V	13–18 months of age	Newly acquired motor skills allow children to experiment and demonstrate the beginning of rational judgment and reasoning. Children further differentiate themselves from objects, understand cause and effect, but have little transfer ability. Children gain spatial awareness (tertiary circular reactions).
VI	18–24 months of age	Preparation for more complex intellectual activities. Children understand object permanence, begin to use language, and engage in domestic mimicry and sex-role behavior. They have some sense of time, but time is exaggerated.

Jean Piaget's theory of cognitive development includes sensorimotor stage (0–24 months of age, broken down in the aforementioned 6 stages) and three additional stages:

Stage	Age	Description
Preoperational	2–7 years of age	From 2–4 years of age, during the preconceptual substage, children use language and symbols, have poor logical ability, and show egocentrism. From 4–7 years of age, during the intuitive substage, children establish a concept of cause and effect, but it may be faulty because of transductive reasoning. They may engage in magical thinking, centration, and animism.
Concrete operational	7–11 years of age	Cause and effect is better understood, and children understand concrete objects and the concept of conservation.
Formal operational	11 years of age–adult	Children exhibit mature thought processes and the ability to think abstractly. Children and young adults can evaluate different possibilities and outcomes.

Psychosocial Development Model

Eric Erikson's psychosocial development model covers the life span, focusing on conflicts at each stage and the virtue that is the outcome of finding a balance in the conflict. The first five stages relate to infancy and childhood and the last three stages to adult-hood, but childhood development affects later adult development:

Stage	Age	Description
Trust vs. mistrust	Birth–1 year of age	Can result in mistrust or faith and optimism.
Autonomy vs. shame/doubt	1–3 years of age	Can lead to doubt and shame or self-control and willpower.
Initiative vs. guilt	3–6 years of age	Can lead to guilt or direction and purpose.
Industry vs. inferiority	6–12 years of age	Can lead to inadequacy and inferiority or competence.
Identify vs. role confusion	12–18 years of age	Can lead to role confusion or devotion and fidelity to others.
Intimacy vs. isolation	Young adulthood	Can lead to lack of close relationships or love and intimacy.
Generativity vs. stagnation	Middle age	Can lead to stagnation or caring and achievements.
Ego integrity vs. despair	Older adulthood	Can lead to despair (failure to accept changes of aging) or wisdom (acceptance).

Theory of Cognitive Dissonance

Leon Festinger's theory of cognitive dissonance states that individuals attempt to escape dissonance and try to avoid inconsistencies between their beliefs and actions. If dissonance occurs, then beliefs and ideas are more likely to change than actions or behavior. Dissonance can be resolved by understanding and attaching less importance to dissonant beliefs, seeking beliefs that are more consonant to outweigh those that are dissonant, or changing beliefs to avoid inconsistencies. Dissonance is especially a concern when the individual is faced with choices and decision-making. Because people want to avoid dissonance, they may avoid individuals or situations in which dissonance occurs. A cognition is considered a piece of knowledge. When faced with dissonance, the person can:

- Change one cognition to match others, or change all to bring them in line.
- Eliminate one cognition, or add more to bring about consonance.
- Alter the importance of cognitions.

Attribution Theory

Bernard Weiner developed the cognitive theory known as **attribution theory**, which focuses on explaining behavior. Weiner suggested that people attempt to attribute cause to behavior, based on three-stages, which include:

- Observing behavior.
- Determining that the behavior is intentional.
- Attributing the behavior to internal or external causes.

According to this theory, there are four factors to which achievement can be attributed:

- Individual effort
- Ability
- Difficulty of task
- Good or bad luck

People often view their own achievement as the result of effort and ability and the achievements of others as the result of luck. By the same token, people may view personal failures as the result of bad luck and the failure of others as the result of lack of effort or ability. Attributions are classified according to three factors:

- Locus of control (internal/external)
- Stability of causes for behavior
- Ability to control causes

Theory of Cognitive Flexibility

The **theory of cognitive flexibility**, focusing on the use of interactive technology, such as computerized programs, was developed by **Rand J. Spiro**, **Paul J. Feltovitch**, and **Richard L. Coulson**. The theory recognizes the complexity and flexibility of learning and suggests that information must be presented in a variety of perspectives and that materials and presentations must be context specific. According to this theory, the primary factor in learning is the ability of the person to construct knowledge. Basic concepts include:

- Providing multiple and varying presentations of content, including technological presentations (computerized) as well as input from instructors or experts, who can facilitate learning.
- Avoiding oversimplification of content and ensuring that information relates to context.
- Building knowledge rather than transferring information. Learners must interact with the material, such as responding to questions or formulating hypotheses based on information presented, to construct their own conclusions.
- Interconnecting instructional sources.

Theory of Multiple Intelligences

Howard Gardner developed the **theory of multiple intelligences**, which states that there are at least seven categories of "intelligence" that people use to comprehend the world and to learn. Gardner proposed that teaching that engages multiple intelligences is more effective than teaching focused primarily on linguistic or logical and mathematical intelligences (those most commonly addressed in education). Students should be assessed to determine the strengths of their personal intelligence, and teaching should address the student's preferences.
- Linguistic intelligence is the ability to use and understand written or spoken language.
- Logical/mathematical intelligence is the ability to use deductive and inductive reasoning, numbers, and abstract thinking.
- Spatial intelligence is the ability to visualize and comprehend spatial dimensions.
- Bodily/kinesthetic intelligence is the ability to control physical action.
- Musical intelligence is the ability to create and appreciate musical forms.
- Interpersonal intelligence is the ability to communicate and establish relationships with others.
- Intrapersonal intelligence is the ability to use self-knowledge and to be self-aware.

Systems Theory

Systems theory is a method to detect ways to connect seemingly unrelated ideas or functions. An underlying principle of systems theory is that all systems have common ways of processing information. By understanding the basic principles of systems theory an individual can detect, understand, and predict most systems environments. This theory is effective since a system is not just a grouping of individual parts, but also an entity of its own. There are two types of systems: natural and designed.
- Natural systems are those that have not been created by human intervention.
- Designed systems may contain hybrids of human created and natural systems.

An important factor of any system is complexity. Complexity refers to the number of parts that are connected, embedded, and entangled with one another. Embedded is defined as one system being completely housed inside another system. Entangled is defined as one system existing only as a part of another system.

Systems theory, developed by **Ludwig von Bertalanffy** in the 1940s, is an approach that considers an entire system holistically rather than focusing on component parts. Bertalanffy believed that all of the elements of a system and their interrelationships need to be understood because all interact to achieve goals; a change in any one element impacts the other elements and alters outcomes. There are five elements in a system:
- Input: This is what goes into a system in terms of energy or materials.
- Throughput: These are the actions that take place in order to transform input.
- Output: This is the result of the interrelationship between input and processes.
- Evaluation: This is monitoring success or failure.
- Feedback: This is information that results from the process and can be used to evaluate the end result.

To achieve desired outcomes, every part of the process must be considered. The individual parts added together do not constitute the whole because viewing the parts separately does not account for the dynamic quality of interaction that takes place.

Family Systems Theory

Murray Bowen's family systems theory suggests that one must look at the person in terms of his or her family unit because the members of a family have different roles and behavioral patterns; thus, a change in one person's behavior affects the others in the family. There are eight interrelated concepts:

- Triangle theory: Two people comprise a basic unit, but when conflict occurs, a third person is drawn into the unit for stability with the resulting dynamic of two supporting one or two opposing one. This, in turn, draws in other triangles.
- Self-differentiation: People vary in their need for external approval.
- Nuclear family patterns: Marital conflict, one spouse dysfunctional, one or more children with problems, and emotional distance constitute some familiar nuclear family patterns.
- Projection within a family: Problems (emotional) are passed from parent to child.
- Transmission (multigenerational): There are small differences in transmission from parent to child.
- Emotional isolation: Reducing or eliminating family contact results in emotional isolation.
- Sibling order: Sibling order can have a profound influence on behavior and development.
- Emotional process (society): Interactions in society result in regressive or progressive social movements.

> ➤ **Review Video:** <u>Bowen Family Systems</u>
> Visit ***mometrix.com/academy*** *and enter* ***Code: 591496***

Complex Adaptive Theory

Complex adaptive theory holds that complex systems are interdisciplinary systems with multiple components or agents that depend on interaction and adaptation as part of learning. Adaptive systems are open systems that are able to adapt readily to changes and problems. The original adaptive theory referred to biology, but the model has expanded to encompass families, communities, and organizations. Interactions tend to be rich and nonlinear with close associates and with much feedback. Interactions are often random rather than planned. Change is often mutual: Agents change, causing the system to change, and the system changes, causing the agents to change. Adaptive systems are dynamic by nature with interdependent agents acting together to bring about change. Adaptive systems that are self-adjusting are able to avoid chaos even though changes may bring them to the brink. Adaptive systems tend to favor effectiveness over efficiency and are less rule-governed than nonadaptive systems.

Change Theory

Change theory was developed by **Kurt Lewin** and modified by **Edgar Schein**. This management theory is based on three stages:

1. **Motivation to change (unfreezing):** Dissatisfaction occurs when goals are not met, but as previous beliefs are brought into question, survival anxiety occurs. Sometimes, however, anxiety about having to learn different strategies causes resistance that can lead to denial, blaming others, and trying to maneuver or bargain without real change.
2. **Desire to change (unfrozen):** Dissatisfaction is strong enough to override defensive actions. The desire to change is strong but must be coupled with identification of needed changes.

3. **Development of permanent change (refreezing):** The new behavior that has developed becomes habitual, often requiring a change in perceptions of self and establishment of new relationships.

Theory of Reasoned Action

The **theory of reasoned action**, developed in 1975 by **Martin Fishbein** and **Icek Ajzen**, is based on the premise that the actions people take voluntarily can be predicted, according to their personal attitude toward the action and their perception of how others will view their doing the action. There are three basic concepts to the theory:
1. **Attitudes:** These are all of the attitudes about an action, and they may be weighted (i.e., some may be more important than others).
2. **Subjective norms:** People are influenced by those in their social realm (e.g., family, friends) and their attitudes toward particular actions. The influence may be weighted (e.g., the attitude of a spouse may carry more weight than the attitude of a neighbor).
3. **Behavioral intention:** The intention to take action is based on weighing attitudes and subjective norms (opinions of others), resulting in a choice to either take an action or avoid an action.

Theory of Planned Behavior

The **theory of planned behavior**, developed by **Icek Ajzen**, evolved from the theory of reasoned action in 1985 when studies showed that behavioral intention does not necessarily result in action. The theory of planned behavior is more successful in predicting behavior. To the basic concepts of attitudes, subjective norms, and behavioral intentions encompassed by the earlier theory, Ajzen added the concept of perceived behavioral control, which relates to the individual's attitudes about self-efficacy and outcomes. Ajzen's theory shows that beliefs are central:
- Behavioral beliefs lead to attitudes toward a behavior or action.
- Normative beliefs lead to subjective norms.
- Control beliefs lead to perceived behavioral control.

All of these beliefs interact to influence intention and action. Basically, this theory relates to the person's confidence, based on beliefs and social influence of others, that he or she can actually do an action and that the outcome of this action will be positive. This theory considers the power of emotions—such as apprehension or fear—when predicting behavior.

Organizational Development (OD) Model of Change

The **organizational development model** (OD) **of change** within an organization works by focusing on the entire culture of the organization rather than trying to change individual behaviors. OD encourages management-worker cooperation and free flowing communication. Its primary goal is to make the whole workplace an excellent environment for everyone to work towards common goals. There are several steps that must take place in order for OD to be beneficial:
- First, the dynamics of the organization are studied and accurately described in a written document.
- Next, a comprehensive strategic plan for problem solving should be carried out.
- Finally, the necessary resources are obtained and the plan is put into place and carried out.

These three comprehensive steps can be further broken down into the following: initial diagnosis, data collection/confrontation, action planning/problem solving, team building, intergroup development, evaluation and follow-up.

Social Exhange Theory

Social exchange theory developed by George C. Homans, John Thibaut, and Harold Kelley, describes communication as an exchange system in which people attempt to negotiate a return on their "investment" in much the same way that people engage in commerce. Those involved in communication seek a balance between investment and return.

Social Penetration Theory

Social penetration theory, developed by Irwin Altman and Dalmas Taylor, describes the manner in which people use communication to develop closeness to others, proceeding from superficial communication to more explicit self-disclosure, which causes vulnerability but allows for a closer relationship.

Spiral of Science Theory

Spiral of science theory, developed by Elisabeth Noelle-Neuman, looks at the role mass media has in influencing communication and suggests that people fear isolation so that they conform to public opinion as espoused by mass media and mute dissent.

Face-Negotiation Theory

Face-negotiation theory developed by Stella Ting-Toomey assumes that all cultures are concerned with maintaining face, and this affects conflict resolution. The theory encompasses the concepts of "positive face" and "negative face" and suggests that people in individualistic cultures are likely to be less compromising than those in collectivist cultures.

Communication Accommodation Theory

Howard Giles developed the **communication accommodation theory (CAT)** to explain why people alter their communication styles. Individuals may practice convergence, modeling the communication style (i.e., accent, dialect, vocabulary) after the other if seeking approval, or may practice divergence, intentionally using differences in communication to emphasize social differences. Components of CAT include the following:
- Context (social and historical) influences communication.
- Accommodative orientation includes three factors: personality, positive or negative feelings, and understanding areas of conflict.
- Immediate communication is affected by social and political states, motivations, goals, convergence, divergence, linguistic choices, and attributions.

George Gerbner developed the **cultivation theory** to explain the effect media, primarily television, have on cultivating ideas and beliefs related more to the media than to the real world. Gerbner believed that media cultivate beliefs that already exist but spread these beliefs through society, thus affecting people's belief systems and perceptions of reality.

Theory of Adult Development

In his **theory of adult development**, **Robert Peck** expanded on Eric Erikson's stages of adult development, believing that there were seven important tasks required during the last two stages of life.

In middle age:
- Mental flexibility vs. mental rigidity
- Valuing wisdom vs. physical powers
- Socializing vs. sexualizing
- Cathectic (libidinal energy) flexibility vs. cathectic impoverishment

Negative outcomes lead to weak relationships, inflexibility, and resistance to change.

Positive outcomes lead to strong relationships, flexibility in lifestyle, and adaptability to change.

In older adulthood:
- Ego differentiation vs. work role preoccupation
- Body transcendence vs. body preoccupation
- Ego transcendence vs. ego preoccupation

Negative outcomes lead to loss of identity after retirement, depression, inability to accept bodily or functional changes, and fear of death.

Positive outcomes lead to meaningful life after retirement, acceptance of bodily or functional changes, acceptance of death, and feeling that life has been good.

Robert Havighurst, in his **theory of adult development**, stated that there were a number of tasks that needed to be accomplished during each stage of development and that remaining active is important. His adult stages reflect stereotypical roles to some degree related to the 1960s when marrying young was more typical than now.

Stage	Tasks
Early adulthood	Tasks include finding a mate, marrying, having children, managing a home, getting started in an occupation or profession, assuming civic responsibility, and finding a congenial social group.
Middle age	Tasks include achieving civic & social responsibility, maintaining an economic standard of living, raising teen-agers & teaching them to be responsible adults, developing leisure activities, accepting physiological changes related to aging, & adjusting to aging of parents.
Older adulthood	Tasks include adjusting to a decrease in physical strength and health, death of a spouse, life in retirement, and reduced income. Other tasks include establishing ties with those in the same age-group (senior citizen's groups/retirees), meeting social and civic obligations, and establishing physical living arrangements that are satisfactory.

Theory of Andragogy

Malcolm Knowles developed the **theory of andragogy** in relation to adult learners, who are more interested in process than in information and content. Knowles outlined some principles of adult learning and typical characteristics of adult learners that an instructor should consider when planning strategies for teaching parents, families, or staff.

Practical & goal-oriented	• Provide overviews or summaries and examples. • Use collaborative discussions with problem-solving exercises. • Remain organized with the goal in mind.
Self-directed	• Provide active involvement, asking for input. • Allow different options toward achieving goals. • Give them responsibilities.
Knowledgeable	• Show respect for their life experiences or education. • Validate their knowledge and ask for feedback. • Relate new material to information with which they are familiar.
Relevancy-oriented	• Explain how information will be applied. • Clearly identify objectives.
Motivated	• Provide certificates of achievement or some type of recognition for achievement.

Bloom's Taxonomy

Bloom's taxonomy developed by **Benjamin Bloom** outlines behaviors that are necessary for learning, and this can apply to health care. The theory describes three types of learning:

<u>Cognitive:</u> (Gaining intellectual skills to master six categories of learning.)
- Knowledge
- Analysis
- Comprehension
- Synthesis
- Application
- Evaluation

<u>Affective:</u> (Recognizing five categories of feelings and values.)
- Receiving phenomena: accepting the need to learn
- Responding to phenomena: taking an active part in care
- Valuing: understanding the value of becoming independent in care
- Organizing values: understanding how surgery or treatment has improved life
- Internalizing values: accepting condition as part of life; being consistent and self-reliant

<u>Psychomotor:</u> (Mastering six motor skills necessary for independence.)
- Perception: uses sensory information to learn tasks
- Set: shows willingness to perform tasks
- Guided response: follows directions
- Mechanism: does specific tasks
- Complex overt response: displays competence in self-care
- Adaptation: modifies procedures as needed
- Origination: creatively deals with problems

Theory of Social Learning

In the 1970s, **Albert Bandura** proposed the **theory of social learning**, in which learning develops from observation, organizing, and rehearsing behavior that has been modeled. Bandura believed that people were more likely to adopt the behavior if they valued the outcomes, if the outcomes had functional value, and if the person modeling had similarities to the learner and was admired because of status. Behavior is the result of observation of behavioral, environmental, and cognitive interactions. There are four conditions required for modeling:

1. **Attention:** The degree of attention paid to modeling depends on many variables (e.g., physical, social, environmental).
2. **Retention:** A person's ability to retain models depends on symbolic coding, creating mental images, organizing thoughts, and rehearsing (mentally or physically).
3. **Reproduction:** The ability to reproduce a model depends on physical and mental capabilities.
4. **Motivation:** Motivation may derive from past performances, rewards, or vicarious modeling.

Lean Six Sigma

Lean-Six Sigma, a method that combines Six-Sigma with concepts of "lean" thinking, focuses process improvement on strategic goals rather than on a project-by-project basis. This type of program is driven by strong senior leadership that establishes long-term goals and strategies. Physicians are an important part of the process and must be included and engaged. The basis of this program is to reduce error and waste within the organization through continuous learning and rapid change. This is especially important in the field of informatics because of the continually evolving nature of information technology and the costs involved in maintaining currency. There are 4 characteristics to Lean-Six Sigma:

- Long term goals with strategies in place for one- to three-year periods.
- Performance improvement as the underlying belief system.
- Cost reduction through quality increase, supported by statistics evaluating the cost of inefficiency.
- Incorporation of improvement methodology, such as DMAIC, PDCA, or other methods.

Rules, Regulations, and Requirements

Standards Related to Computerized and Information Systems

The Joint Commission has described the need for computer system **standards** in the following areas:
- Access to databases that are located outside the organization and used to compare information, need to be supported and secured.
- Patient confidentiality related to personal health information (PHI) and data security must be ensured.
- Knowledge-based systems should be developed and promoted to allow resident organizational expertise to be used throughout the organization.
- A means to link physician information systems while protecting patient privacy and data security.
- Projects that are designed to achieve quality improvements should be supported.
- Data integrity and overall system security must be ensured.
- Procedural controls that are currently in place for documentation should be integrated into the new computerized standards.
- A regular assessment of needs and system capacity for growth should be supported.

The Joint Commission outlined factors it believes are important for **information standards**:
- Measures must be adopted that are designed to protect an individual's personal health information. This may be accomplished by limiting access to information based on a user's need to know, having strict policies regarding the removal of records, and making sure data is physically and electronically safeguarded.
- A national standard for data entry should be created and followed. All users should be trained both in system use and information management. Educational courses may include lectures on how information that is entered into a computer system is transformed into data that can later be used to perform statistical analysis and support decision-making.
- All information should be available both on the computer and in print form.

> ➤ **Review Video:** The Joint Commission Core Principles
> *Visit **mometrix.com/academy** and enter **Code: 676427***

Centers for Medicare and Medicaid Services

The **Centers for Medicare and Medicaid Services (CMS)** maintain a list of approved accreditation organizations for health care providers, as providers and suppliers who have been accredited by one of these national accrediting agencies are exempt from state surveys in determining if they are in compliance with Medicare-mandated conditions. Approved organizations include the Joint Commission, Community Health Association Program, and the Accreditation Commission for Health Care. The CMS has established an incentive program for adoption, upgrade, or use of electronic health records (EHRs). Those applying for incentive programs must use certified EHR systems that demonstrate that they can store and share patient data securely. Health care providers who are eligible for incentive pay from Medicare or Medicaid can receive up to $44,000 over a 5-year period, while eligible hospitals and critical access hospitals can receive a beginning base payment of $2 million. Medicare eligibility guidelines and Medicaid eligibility guidelines vary for both eligible professionals and eligible hospitals.

Updating Documentation Requirements Based on Changes to Regulatory or Accreditation Standards

The nursing informatics specialist must **update documentation requirements based on changes to regulatory or accreditation standards**. This means that the nurse must be cognizant of accreditation standards, such as those by the Joint Commission, and current regulations, such as those related to the Centers for Medicare and Medicaid Services (CMS) or the Health Insurance Portability and Accountability Act, which must be monitored closely to determine if current documentation is adequate and what changes must be made. Accreditation standards require huge amounts of paperwork to demonstrate compliance, so building requirements into the system can save time when reports are due; thus, the nursing informatics specialist must consider the need to retrieve data as well as document necessary information when updating. While CMS provides updates regarding most federal regulations, states may have additional requirements that must be accommodated. Changes should be done well in advance of required compliance so that staff members can become familiar with changes, and problems with changes can be evaluated.

Accredited Standards Committee and the Pharmacy Standards Association

These organizations have created universal standards for healthcare computerized tasks in the United States. The goal is to create records that are more accurate, avoid duplication, and ensure communication between computer systems.

- The Accredited Standards Committee (ASC) created the standards associated with administrative medical insurance tasks. The current version, X12N, is used nationwide. X12N helps with claims, enrollment, and determining insurance eligibility.
- The National Council for Prescription Drug Programs (NCPDP) develops pharmacy standards for the U.S. Electronic claims processing under this standard was first introduced in 1992 and has gone on to make up nearly 100% of retail pharmacy claims being processed in real-time. Healthcare providers send EDI (electronic prescriptions) messages to the pharmacy directly. Another NCPCP set of standards, HL7, focuses on the communication of information within and between different healthcare facilities. Collaboration between X12N and HL7 has resulted in the EHR-S (electronic health record system) standards as a way to solidify all aspects of patient healthcare under a single system.

> **Review Video:** Prescription Authenticity
> *Visit mometrix.com/academy and enter Code:* **245184**

> **Review Video:** Prescription Labels
> *Visit mometrix.com/academy and enter Code:* **339257**

Maximizing Reimbursement

Methods to maximize reimbursement include:
- Recording of information and sending of claims in a timely manner.
- Using care managers to determine the most cost-effective care plan.
- Using standardized billing codes (Current Procedural Terminology, International Classification of Diseases [ICD]).
- Ensuring that the health care provider's National Provider Identifier is present on all claims.

- Updating systems promptly when new coding (e.g., ICD-10) and billing regulations (e.g., pay-for-performance) are issued rather than waiting for the end of the grace period so that problems can be identified and corrected early.
- Ensuring that the presentation on admission (Medicare severity diagnosis-related group code) diagnosis is correct to avoid a different discharge diagnosis.
- Monitoring quality of care to prevent complications and reduce costs related to the do-not-pay list.
- Sending claims in the correct form and to the correct address for different entities: insurance companies, Medicaid, and Medicare.

Pay-for-Performance or Value-Based Purchasing

A reimbursement system called **pay-for-performance (P4P)** or **value-based purchasing**, one element of the Affordable Care Act of 2010, is an alternative to standard pay-for-care reimbursement. Some states, such as California, have P4P plans in effect, and Medicare also has a number of P4P initiatives and demonstration projects. The primary objective of P4P programs is to reward health care providers when patients have good results (e.g., discharge within a defined period without complications), although there remains some controversy regarding measuring quality performance. Payment is related to quality rather than quantity of service, so ongoing quality improvement processes must be in place to maximize reimbursement. In some cases, bonus incentives may be provided. Disincentives, such as reduced payment for never events (inexcusable outcomes), are also considered. There are both hospital-based P4P plans and physician-based P4P plans.

Present-on-Admission Medicare Severity Diagnosis-Related Group

On admission to acute hospitals under the Medicare Inpatient Prospective Payment System (IPPS), patients must be given a **present-on-admission (POA) Medicare severity diagnosis-related group (MS-DRG)** diagnosis. The MS-DRG should include primary and secondary diagnoses present during the admission process. This is a concern regarding maximizing reimbursement because hospital-acquired conditions may not be covered if there is a change at discharge from the POA diagnosis. A POA indicator must be on all claims:
- Y: Medicare pays for a condition if a hospital-acquired condition (HAC) is present on admission.
- N: Medicare will not pay for condition if a HAC is present on discharge but not on admission.
- U: Medicare will not pay for condition if a HAC is present and documentation is not adequate to determine if the condition was present on admission.
- W: Medicare will pay for condition if a HAC is present and if the health care provider cannot determine if the condition was present on admission.

Do-Not-Pay List

As a means to control quality of care and to cut costs, Medicare instituted a **do-not-pay list** for serious, preventable, hospital-acquired conditions and complications for which Medicare will not reimburse hospitals; thus, avoiding these complications is a critical element in maximizing reimbursement and requires ongoing monitoring of quality care and staff education. Additionally, some insurance companies are following suit, so this has the potential to impact reimbursement seriously. For example, if surgery is done on the wrong side or botched, Medicare will not pay the costs. If a blood clot occurs after hip replacement surgery, Medicare will not pay for treatment. There are currently over forty categories on the do-not-pay list, including the following:

- Fall or other trauma that causes serious injury.
- Stages III and IV pressure ulcers.
- Vascular catheter-associated infections.
- Catheter-associated urinary tract infections.
- Transfusion reaction from blood incompatibility.
- Postoperative dehiscence.
- Surgical deaths associated with treatable serious complications.

Malpractice and Negligence

Risk management must attempt to determine the burden of proof for acts of **negligence**, including compliance with duty, breaches in procedures, degree of harm, and cause as a finding of negligence can lead to a **malpractice** suit. Negligence indicates that proper care, based on established standards, has not been provided. State regulations regarding negligence may vary, but all have some statutes of limitation. There are a number of different types of negligence.

- Negligent conduct indicates that an individual failed to provide reasonable care or to protect/assist another, based on standards and expertise.
- Gross negligence is willfully providing inadequate care while disregarding the safety and security of another.
- Contributory negligence involves the injured parties contributing to the harm done.
- Comparative negligence attempts to determine what percentage of negligence is attributed to each individual involved.

Liability

With the marked increase in use of electronic health records (EHRs) has come increased concern regarding **liability** because the EHR documents all actions in real time. For example, if there is a delay between the time a patient event occurs and when the health care provider responds, the duration of time is documented in the record and cannot be altered. This can give the appearance of negligence even if the delay was unavoidable. Additionally, errors tend to increase with any major change, and there is a learning curve in adjusting to new technology, so information may be entered into EHRs incorrectly and a facility may be liable if it did not provide adequate staff education. Providers used to reports on paper may not access electronic reports in a timely manner. Hardware or software incompatibilities may cause information, such as medicine orders, to be altered or deleted. If health care providers provide patients access to them via e-mail or messaging and do not respond promptly to those messages, then they may be liable for malpractice.

Patient Data Misuse

Patient data misuse is an increasing problem with the rapid proliferation of electronic health records (EHRs). Types of misuse include:

- Identity theft: Health records often contain identifying information, such as Social Security numbers, credit card numbers, birthdates, and addresses, making patients vulnerable.
- Unauthorized access: Although EHRs and computerized documentation systems are password protected, providers sometimes share passwords or unwittingly expose their passwords when logging in, inadvertently allowing access to information about patients.

- Privacy violations: Even professionals authorized to access a patient's record may share private information with others, such as family or friends.
- Security breaches: Data are vulnerable to security breaches because of careless, inadequate security, especially when various business associates, such as billing companies, have access to private information.

Proprietary Data

Propriety data derive from proprietary software that has been developed internally or used under contract with a company, such as Cisco, which developed the software. Proprietary software should be protected by patent or copyright and use restricted to protect intellectual property, such as patient lists, financial reports, or details about an organization. Those who use proprietary software should require that all those working with the data, including third parties, sign a nondisclosure agreement to prevent information regarding the software or data from being stolen or misused. Stealing proprietary data is common when people leave an organization and is often used to benefit a new employer; however, stealing legally protected information is an act of fraud. Security experts should constantly monitor software and data to ensure that they have not been invaded by malware (malicious software), which can steal information, damage systems, or disrupt operations.

Privacy and Security Rules

The Health Insurance Portability and Accountability Act of 1996 mandates **privacy** and **security rules** (Code of Federal Regulations, Title 45, part 164) to ensure that health information and individual privacy are protected.
- Privacy rule: Protected information includes any information included in the medical record (electronic or paper), conversations between the physician and other health care providers, billing information, and any other form of health information. Procedures must be in place to limit access and disclosures.
- Security rule: Any electronic health information must be secure and protected against threats, hazards, or nonpermitted disclosures, in compliance with established standards. Implementation specifications must be addressed for any adopted standards. Administrative, physical, and technical safeguards must be in place as well as policies/procedures to comply with standards. Security requirements include: limiting access to those authorized, use of unique identifiers for each user, automatic logoff, encryption and decryption of protected health care information, authentication that health care data have not been altered or destroyed, monitoring of logins, and security of transmission. Access controls must include a unique identifier, procedures to access the system in emergencies, time out, and encryption/decryption.

Security of Patient Information

The Joint Commission outlined many factors that it believes are important to the **security of patient information**. The two major factors are:

1. **Information should be transmitted accurately and quickly**. This includes the following:
   - Requested information should be supplied within 24 of the request. It should be transmitted in whatever format the user needs.
   - Orders should be put in place with as little delay as possible and test results should be entered into the system quickly.

- 27 -

- Errors should be minimized. This could be achieved with the implementation of a computerized system such as a pharmacy system.
- Methods of communication should be evaluated for efficiency.

2. **Clinical and non-clinical systems should be fully integrated**. This includes the following:
- Records should be customizable to the patient and their individual needs.
- The system should be able to create reports based on the user's demands.
- Comparisons between healthcare organizations should be fully supported.

Health Insurance Portability and Accountability Act (HIPAA)

The **Health Insurance Portability and Accountability Act** (HIPAA) was passed in 1996 to protect patient privacy rights. This is especially important given the large amount of sensitive data that is now handled electronically through large databases. Some key compliance dates for HIPAA are listed below (for large health plans):
- October 16, 2002: Electronic transactions and code sets are to be identified.
- April 14, 2003: Privacy standards are to be set.
- July 30, 2004: Standards for employer identification are to be set.
- April 21, 2005: Standards for system and data security are to set.
- May 23, 2007: Standards for provider identification are to be set.

These uniform standards will allow the data repositories of large healthcare systems to be efficiently monitored for adherence to the HIPAA regulations, thus assuring patient rights to privacy are honored.

The **Health Insurance Portability and Accountability Act** (HIPAA) establishes standards for computer-based record keeping in the healthcare industry. Timetables were established that included fines for noncompliance by certain dates. This legislation required the Director of Health and Human Services (DHHS) to create:
- Rules regarding how electronic transactions are processed.
- A unique identification code for all providers, health plans, and employers.
- A way to keep patient information secure and private.

The Health Insurance Portability and Accountability Act also granted certain rights to patients including the right to view their own medical records and request that corrective changes are made to their medical files. A key attribute of HIPAA is that healthcare providers may not keep personal health information (PHI) unprotected on their computer systems.

In order for a healthcare organization to comply with the **Health Insurance Portability and Accountability Act,** they should evaluate their system's **compliance** on a frequent basis. The following is a list of questions that should be asked during the evaluation procedure:
- Where is patient data stored?
- Does each user have a unique sign-on that must be entered before gaining access to the system?
- Are workstations physically secured (e.g., in a locked room)?
- Does the system have an auto-log off function?
- Is the system safe from unauthorized users?

- Is all hardware and software up to date?
- Where are backup devices kept?
- Are print copies of information disposed of properly (e.g., shredded)?

Privacy and Confidentiality

Patient **privacy** and **confidentiality** are two main concerns especially as they apply to the collection and storage of computer records. Patients have a right to privacy and that any information they choose to share is only accessible to authorized personnel.

- Privacy is defined as "freedom from intrusion, or control over the exposure of self or personal information." In healthcare, an individual's right to privacy includes remaining anonymous by request, deciding what information is collected, and how that information is used.
- Confidentiality is the careful sharing of private information to people who have a valid interest in helping the individual. The ethical duty of confidentiality requires the information to be stored or transferred in a secure way. The individual's right to decide how information is shared is known as information privacy. This includes the right to accurate information being collected and stored. Information security includes the measures taken to ensure that records are kept accurate and are not accessible to unauthorized people.

> ➤ **Review Video:** <u>Confidentiality</u>
> Visit *mometrix.com/academy* and enter *Code:* **250384**

System Penetration

System penetration occurs when someone other than the authorized system personnel access a private computer system. System penetration can lead to lost time and money in addition to negative public relations. Losing private information has become a regular headline in the news. In today's world of cyber criminals, the robbery of personal information from a computer system is a far larger threat than physical breaking and entering. There are typically three types of people who attempt system penetration: opportunists, hackers, and information specialists. Opportunists are those individuals who have valid access to a computer system and use the information stored there for nefarious purposes. Hackers may see system security as a challenge to rise to and attempt system penetration for the thrill. Similar to hackers, an information specialist is someone who has been trained to work with computers on a professional level, but then uses this training to commit crimes.

Sabotage, Errors, and Disasters

Sabotage: The willful destruction of computer equipment (or database records) is defined as sabotage. The majority of these types of acts are committed by angry or unhappy employees. The others are caused by external hackers to the system who destroy (or erase) records for their own notoriety.

Errors: There are several ways that errors occur in computer systems: poor design, incorrect data entry, or retrieval of an incorrect entry. It is important that when errors are found, they be reported to the system administrator immediately.

Disasters: A disaster may cause the system to be shut down entirely for an undefined length of time. For this reason, it is important to have backup procedures (both manual and at a remote site) in place and to conduct practice drills regularly so that the entire operation will not be put at risk.

Unauthorized User

While system access by an external hacker is a valid concern, the biggest security problem for health database systems is the **unauthorized user**. An unauthorized user is an employee of the company that has legitimate access to the database system, but access of information beyond what is needed for their job or task. This type of individual purposefully or inadvertently views data that they should not, creates a disruption in the availability of information, or corrupts the integrity of the stored data. Under HIPAA regulations, all healthcare facilities must guarantee patient information privacy under penalty of law. Because healthcare databases may be very large and fragmented, it is sometimes difficult to restrict an employee's access to only those patients (or specific patient test results) to which they have a valid need to access.

Malicious Programs

There are five types of **malicious computer programs**:

Viruses
- Can damage data, but may only be an annoyance.
- Computer must be running in order for these to spread.

Worms
- Named after the pattern of damage they perform.
- Use LAN and WAN practices to spread and reproduce.

Trojan horses
- Appear to be performing a legitimate task, but actually do something else.
- May look like a regular system login, but in fact records information, which it then sends back to its creator for malicious reasons.
- Do not self-replicate.
- Easily confined once found.

Logic bombs
- Triggered by a specific bit of data.
- Can be hidden in a normal program.
- Type of virus.

Bacteria
- Type of virus.
- Are not attached to existing programs.

Avoiding the Installation of Malicious Software

In order to avoid **malicious software** (such as viruses or Trojan horses), use the following proven methods:
- Monitor and verify that only licensed software is uploaded into the system.
- Make sure that all network computers have updated virus detection software installed and that it is set-up to make daily scans of the entire system.
- Be wary of e-mail and never open a file attachment from an unfamiliar source.

- Keep copies of computer start-up files, original software, work files, and directory structure in case problems arise. Keep a list of where each piece of hardware or software was purchased, the date of purchase, and all serial numbers in a secure location separate from the system.
- Update software regularly to fix security vulnerabilities.
- Finally, be sure that all staff members are familiar with the appropriate use of software, hardware, and e-mail.

Antivirus Software and Spyware

Two types of programs are essential to the security of today's computers:
- **Antivirus software**: New computer viruses are being developed and detected all the time, making it necessary to have antivirus software that is completely updated. Many vendors of antivirus software allow the user to purchase updates for a small fee. These updates are generally downloaded from the company's website using an internet connection. The software then should be scheduled to check for viruses on a regular basis (typically daily).
- **Spyware detection software**: Spyware is a type of software that implants itself into a computer system and sends information back to its maker. Spyware is typically attached to many "free" software programs available for download on the internet. All computers connected to the internet are at risk to spyware. Therefore, updated spyware detection software should be run regularly to find and eradicate these programs.

Computer Security Mechanisms

Keeping computer systems safe requires a mixture of both physical and electronic **security**. This consists of:
- Physical security may be maintained by placing computers or servers in restricted areas. Laptop and other portable computers should be fitted with locks or alarms and have extensive password protection in place.
- Since many systems are open to remote access, it is important that even if they are physically secure that they have electronic protection also. Firewalls help protect systems from unauthorized access by presenting an electronic barrier between the system and the remote user. A firewall is able to look at incoming information and only let through that which is approved. Firewalls may also be placed within a system to keep parts of it off limits to individuals who are authorized users of the system in general. It is a good practice to use a firewall to protect such things as payroll, personnel data, and client information.

Encryption

Patient information that is stored in databases is of a sensitive and confidential nature. Therefore, it is a requirement to use **encryption** when transmitting this information to other locations. Encryption is the process of using mathematical formulas to code data so that it is unrecognizable if it is intercepted by someone outside of the system. There are three distinct ways that encryption can be handled by a company: at the desktop, administrated, or server-wide. When an employee encrypts messages at their desktop, it protects the message, but unfortunately may also hide information (such as viruses) from detection by the system administrator. A company may also assign an encryption administrator to handle the coding and decoding of messages. With today's computer systems, the most effective way to encrypt messages is to have the central server encrypt every outgoing message automatically. This requires no manual procedures whatsoever.

Authentication Security

There are three levels of user **authentication security** scaled to the amount of security offered (e.g., Level Three offers the most security):

Level One
- Once an individual is logged into the system (using their name and password), their name appears on the screen and their access is tracked as they use the system.
- Users are automatically logged out after some period of inactivity and must login again to continue using the system.
- Must update their password (set to a specific level of complexity) on a regular basis (e.g., monthly).

Level Two
- Encrypted key-based authentication.
- User must present computer access card (CAC) to the system before they can log on.
- Automatic log out if CAC is too far from the computer.

Level Three
- Biometric authentication: Uses something unique to the individual such as: fingerprint, retinal scan, or face recognition. Some newer laptops now come with a fingerprint scanner built-in.
- Cannot be lost or stolen.

Secure Passwords

The following is a list of recommendations for creating **secure passwords** on a computer system:
- Common guidance for password selection is to use at least eight characters and have a combination of character types (uppercase, lowercase, symbols, and numbers). However, many experts have concluded that a long password (20+ characters) is more secure than a complex short password.
- Each application should have its own password. That is, a separate password for each application that the user is authorized to access.
- Use a password security tester to be sure the password is strong enough. This program will attempt to "break" a given password and determine how effective it is.
- Never save passwords on the internet browser. Disable the "save form data" option in the privacy settings. Also, never access the computer system from a public computer (such as those found in a library).
- Do not use personal identifiers such as social security numbers, birthdays, or names.
- Do not write passwords down.
- Have a set expiry time limit for passwords and do not allow them to be repeated.

Audit Trails

Audit trails are records of activity related to systems and applications, users' access, and use of systems and applications. One system may employ a number of different audit trails. Audit trails are a security tool that allows administrators to track individual users, identify the cause of problems, note data modification and misuse of equipment, and reconstruct computer events. Audit trails can also indicate penetration or attempted penetration. Audit trails include event records and keystroke monitoring, which shows each keystroke entered by a user and the electronic response.

- Audit trails at the system level generally record any logins, including identification, date, and time, devices used, and functions.
- Audit trails at the application level monitor activity within the application, including opened files, editing, reading, deleting, and printing.

Audit trails for users include all activities by the user, such as commands, accessed files, and deletions.

Tokens

Tokens are items used to authenticate a person's identity and allow access to a system. They commonly require the use of not only the token but also a personal identification number or user name and password. Some devices, such as the SecureID token by RSA generate one-time passwords. Tokens may be in the form of access cards, which may use different technologies: photos, optical-coding, electric circuits, and magnetic strips. They may also be contained in common objects, such as a key fob. Some tokens must be plugged directly into the computer. Different types of tokens include:

- **ID cards**: These include driver's licenses and employee badges but provide very little security as they can easily be falsified or stolen.
- **Challenge-response tokens**: These combine use of the token with user information, such as user name and password.
- **Smart cards**: These contain microchips with information that can be programmed to allow access, like a debit card.

Typically, databases track who is accessing a system and the duration of access.

Security Failures

Security failures may occur as the result of a number of different problems.

- **System penetration**: Penetration can result from undetected vulnerabilities. Penetration tests should be conducted to identify vulnerabilities. Perpetrators may be cyberhackers, hackers, computer specialists, authorized users, unauthorized users, and opportunists.
- **Destruction/sabotage**: This includes physical damage to the system or purposeful alterations in applications. Perpetrators may be anyone who has access to the computer system or who has issues with management or other aspects of the organization.
- **Mistakes/errors**: Errors may result from poor design; incorrect entries; system changes; poorly trained personnel; and absence of adequate procedures, policies, and education.
- **Password management**: Poor management procedures, such as sharing passwords or posting user names and passwords where they can be accessed by unauthorized persons, can allow unauthorized people to access a system.
- **Device compromise**: Handheld devices, such as personal digital assistants and smart phones, are vulnerable to theft and can easily transmit viruses and worms.

Physical Security

Physical security is essential for computer systems. The first step is to determine who has access to different types of equipment and then to apply methods to limit access to only those authorized through use of user names and passwords or tokens. Servers should be rack-mounted in locked, climate-controlled rooms that have regular surveillance. Vulnerable devices should remain in the locked room. Data should be backed up routinely and stored or archived in a secure remote location. Workstations should be secure, including printers. Cable lock systems should be used to secure equipment, including laptops, to furniture. Operating systems should be locked when not in use, and encryption software should be used to secure routers that are used for wireless transmission. Equipment should be in restricted areas. Remote access should be done with secure modems and encryption. Public access to the internet should be on a different network from that used to transmit health care information.

Device Access Control

Device access control can encompass a wide range of technologies and procedures. The first step is to determine what class of users has access to different devices and then what method of authentication (e.g., password, biometrics) for role and entity-based access is required. Clear policies and procedures must be in place for both access and use of devices. Role and entity-based access should be determined by the individual role and function within the organization rather than on hierarchy. Networked medical devices and information technology devices may be on the same network, and handheld devices may connect to multiple networks; thus, these situations pose additional security risks. All handheld devices, which pose the most risk, must be password protected. Security of access control must be strictly enforced, and those who violate security policies and procedures should have restricted use. Each potential device user must be correctly identified and access controlled. Commercial access control programs are available for health care organizations.

Time-Outs

Once a person has logged in and gained access to a computer, the computer is vulnerable if that user leaves the computer and fails to log out, so computers connected to a secure system routinely have a **time-out** feature (automatic log off) that locks the system after a prescribed period (usually 10–15 minutes) in which there is no mouse or keyboard activity. Some software programs and applications also have time-out features. Once the time out is initiated, a person must log in again in the prescribed manner to gain access. Time out/automatic logoff is one of the security procedures that must be addressed for part of the Health Insurance Portability and Accountability Act's security rule. The users' workflow and type of use of devices should be considered when scheduling automatic log off.

Major Threats to Computer Systems

There are **four main categories of threat** to a computer system. These threats can incapacitate a computer system for a short or very long time, depending on their severity:
- **Environmental disasters** can be either natural or man-made. Natural disasters include blizzards, earthquakes, epidemics, floods, tornadoes, and hurricanes. Man-made environmental disasters include: chemical contamination, power outages, accidents when hardware is being transported, and toxic fumes.
- **Human error** is one of the major causes of problems with a computer system. Human error includes overwriting files, accidentally deleting files, and overloading the system with unnecessary programs.

- **Human mischief** includes theft, malicious programs, terrorism, and cybercrime. Since the attacks of September 11, 2001, organizations have also had to include potential loss of large numbers of information system employees in their disaster planning scenarios.
- **Equipment failure** includes disconnected wiring, CPU crashes, and storage drive failure.

Health Information Technology for Economic and Clinical Health Act

The American Recovery and Reinvestment Act of 2009 included the **Health Information Technology for Economic and Clinical Health Act (HITECH)**. HITECH provides incentive payments to Medicare practitioners (usually physicians) to adopt electronic health records (EHRs). EHRs must be certified and meet the requirement for "meaningful use." Additionally, HITECH provides penalties in the form of reduced Medicare payments for those who do not adopt EHRs, unless exempted by hardship (e.g., rural practices). Security provisions include the following:
- Individuals and Health and Human Services must be notified of a breach in security of personal health information.
- Business partners must meet security regulations or face penalties.
- The sale or marketing of personal health information is restricted.
- Individuals must have access to electronic health information.
- Individuals must be informed of disclosures of personal health information.

HITECH also provides matching grants to institutes of higher education and funding for training for health information technology, promotes research and development of health information technology, and provides grants to the Indian Health Services for adoption of health internet technology.

Ethical Principles

International Council of Nurses (ICN) Code of Ethics

The following is an outline of the ICN (International Council of Nurses) **Code of Ethics** for nurses in regards to **patients**:

- Foremost, the nurse's responsibility is to the patient. The patient must receive the best possible care and their rights and well-being are respected and maintained.
- Respect and support patient rights, religious beliefs, values, and customs. The patient should be able to live their way of life while under care. This means that they should be allowed to follow their culture and traditions as best as possible.
- Make sure the patient gives informed consent for any treatment. The patient has the ultimate say as to whether or not they receive treatment. The right of the patient to accept or refuse a given treatment through the informed consent process is essential.
- Keep patient information confidential. The patient's right to privacy is protected under law and should be respected.

In addition, nurses should be proponents for community health and act to promote environmentalism.

The International Council of Nurses (ICN) has developed a **Code of Ethics** for nurses in regards to **coworkers**. Healthcare is a team-oriented process with all attention focused on the well-being of the patient. Effective interaction with other team members (coworkers) is a key to success in this environment. The following bullet points are key areas that need attention:

- Keep relationships with coworkers cooperative and professional.
- Make sure that patients are safe and promptly deal with unprofessional or dangerous conduct on the part of coworkers.
- Take care not to delegate more work than the individual is able to handle.
- Promote continuing education in the workplace.
- Keep the lines of communication open between departments, management, etc.

> ➤ **Review Video:** Organizational Ethics
> *Visit **mometrix.com/academy** and enter **Code: 885880***

This is an area that needs constant monitoring by workers and management. Any drift from optimal conditions should be addressed before the patient is exposed to any negative effects of poor teamwork.

The following is an outline of the International Council of Nurses (ICN) **Code of Ethics** for nurses in regards to **practice and profession**:

- Keep up to date with the practice of nursing through continuing education. This entails taking continuing education courses and adding certifications to one's resume.
- Look after one's own health in order to maintain quality of care to the patient. It is very easy to forget about taking care of yourself while working with sick patients on long shifts. The importance of keeping healthy is a key to providing excellent care to patients.
- Do not take on more than can be reasonably handled. In the current cost cutting healthcare environment, nurses are being asked to do more with less. This can lead to burn out and high staff turnover.
- Uphold a high standard of personal conduct.

- Make sure that all new applications of technology are safe for use in treatment and do not compromise the dignity of the patient.
- Develop and put in place ethical standards in clinical, management, education, and research.

Nursing Code of Ethics

The American Nurses Association developed the **Nursing Code of Ethics**. There are nine provisions, which are listed below:
- The nurse treats all individuals with respect and consideration, regardless of social circumstances or health condition.
- The nurse's primary commitment is to the individual regardless of conflicts that may arise.
- The nurse promotes and advocates for the individual's health, safety, and rights, maintaining privacy and confidentiality and protecting him or her from questionable practices or care.
- The nurse is responsible for his or her own care practices and determines appropriate delegation of care.
- The nurse must retain respect for self and his or her own integrity and competence.
- The nurse participates in ensuring that the health care environment is conducive to providing good health care that is consistent with professional and ethical values.
- The nurse participates in education and knowledge development to advance the profession.
- The nurse collaborates with others to promote efforts to meet health needs.
- The nursing profession articulates values and promotes and maintains the integrity of the profession.

International Medical Informatics Association Code of Ethics

The **International Medical Informatics Association Code of Ethics** was developed in 2002 and recently revised. Part I, the introduction, includes the six primary ethical principles: autonomy (self-determination), equality and justice (equal treatment), beneficence (promoting good), nonmalfeasance (preventing harm), impossibility (predicated on possibility), and integrity (honesty and diligence). General principles in the introduction include the following:
- The right to privacy, regarding sharing of personal information and control of collection, methods of collection, and storage.
- Open process of data collection with patient informed.
- Security of all data collection and protection from data manipulation.
- Right to access of personal data.
- Legitimate infringement or the consideration for greater good of society in regard to individual's right to privacy.
- Infringement of right to privacy with minimum interference
- Accountability for infringement.

Part II, rules of ethical conduct, includes subject-centered duties, duties toward health care professionals, duties toward institutions and employers, duties toward society, self-regarding duties, and professional duties.

Promoting an Environment for Ethical Decision-Making and Patient Advocacy

An environment for ethical decision-making and **patient advocacy** does not appear when it is needed; it requires planning and preparation. The expectation for the institution should clearly communicate that nurses are legally and morally responsible for assuring competent care and respecting the rights of patients and other stakeholders. Decisions regarding ethical issues often must be made quickly with little time for contemplation; therefore, ethical issues that may arise should be identified and discussed. Clearly defined procedures and policies for dealing with conflicts, including an active ethics committee, in-service training, and staff meetings, must be established. Patients and families need to be part of the ethical environment, which means empowering them by providing patient/family information (e.g., print form, video, audio) that outlines patient's rights and procedures for expressing their wishes and dealing with ethical conflicts. Respect for privacy and confidentiality and a nonpunitive atmosphere are essential.

Policies and Procedures

Development of Policies

The **development of policies** must be based on best practices and conform to state, federal, and accreditation regulations and guidelines. Empowerment includes encouraging participation of all staff in policy making. Objectives for policies should be clearly outlined. In some cases, policies may be broad and cover all aspects of an organization, but in other cases, policies may be much more specific, such as a policy regarding use of computer equipment. Conflict of interest policies should be in place to ensure that those involved in review activities should not be primary caregivers or have an economic or personal interest in a case under review. Policies should ensure that access to protected health information be limited to those who need the information to complete duties related to direct care or performance improvement review activities. Policy and procedure manuals should be readily available organization-wide in easily accessible format, such as online. Policy issues may include cost-effectiveness, insurance coverage, criteria for qualified staff, and legal implications.

Review of Informatics Policies and Procedures

Review of informatics policies and **procedures** should be done in response to surveillance/evaluation reports, as policies and procedures should be written with clear goals and outcomes in mind. A comprehensive review should include:
- **Analysis of achievement of goals:** If goals are met or exceeded, then new goals may need to be set. If goals are not met, then policies, procedures, or training were either inadequate or unrealistic.
- **Analysis of variances and assessing risk factors.**
- **Staff input:** Meetings to discuss adequacy or problems with current policies and procedures can be held to gather opinions of staff. In addition, cross-sectional questionnaires regarding compliance, knowledge, and training can be used
- **Training review:** Training should be ongoing and coupled with clear expectations of staff compliance.

Administrative Computer Related Policies

A healthcare facility must have a **policy** regarding computer system use. This policy should be discussed during the orientation process and before the employee is allowed to access the computer system. The policy should outline the regulations pertaining to client confidentiality, ethical use of computers, and the disciplinary actions that will be taken against employees who do not adhere to the policy. Many organizations insist that staff members sign an agreement (which states that system misuse can result in disciplinary action) before system access instructions. System access is usually achieved by entering a user name and password. Security measures may include setting the complexity of the password and the password change intervals.

Downtime Forms

Downtime forms are used for record-keeping when the information system has scheduled or unscheduled downtime. Policies should be in place stating when use of downtime forms should begin (often after 1 hour). Downtime forms should be readily available at the point of care and correspond as much as possible to the screen presentations in the information system so that information can be easily entered when the system is back up. Screenshots may provide helpful guides when creating downtime forms but are usually not flexible enough for accurate record-keeping. Each department may have different downtime forms, depending on functions. Some systems have print options for forms, and these should be preprinted and ready for use. Forms should be up-to-date and contain correct coding (e.g., current procedural terminology codes) when applicable. Print medication records should contain allergy information.

Communication Skills Needed for Leading Intra- and Interdisciplinary Teams

A number of **communication skills** are needed to lead and facilitate coordination of **intra-** and **interdisciplinary teams**, such as the following:

- Communicating openly is essential with all members encouraged to participate as valued members of a cooperative team.
- Avoiding interrupting or interpreting the point another is trying to make allows free flow of ideas.
- Avoiding jumping to conclusions as this can effectively shut off communication.
- Active listening requires paying attention and asking questions for clarification rather than challenging the ideas of others.
- Respecting the opinions and ideas of others, even when they are opposed to one's own, is absolutely essential.
- Reacting and responding to facts rather than feelings allows one to avoid angry confrontations or diffuse anger.
- Clarifying information or opinions stated can help avoid misunderstandings.
- Keeping unsolicited advice out of the conversation shows respect for others and allows them to solicit advice without feeling pressured.

Teambuilding

Leading, facilitating, and participating in performance improvement teams requires a thorough understanding of the dynamics of **team building:**

- **Initial interactions:** This is the time when members begin to define their roles and develop relationships, determining if they are comfortable in the group.
- **Power issues:** The members observe the leader and determine who controls the meeting and how control is exercised, beginning to form alliances.
- **Organizing:** Methods to achieve work are clarified and team members begin to work together, gaining respect for each other's contributions and working toward a common goal.
- **Team identification:** Interactions often become less formal as members develop rapport, and members are more willing to help and support each other to achieve goals.
- **Excellence:** This develops through a combination of good leadership, committed team members, clear goals, high standards, external recognition, spirit of collaboration, and a shared commitment to the process.

Workgroup Formation

A **workgroup** is a small number of people working together toward a common goal. An advantage of working in groups is that the environment allows for increased insight and creativity. A disadvantage is that workgroups sometimes fail because members of the group allow personal conflicts (in terms of personality and work styles) to interfere with the group's goal. A popular concept identifies four stages in group development:

Forming – This is where a group is formed and the members begin to get to know one another. Typically, individuals are quiet and polite to one another.
Storming – This is the stage where conflicts normally arise. Effective communications must be occurring.

Norming – Typically, conflicting factions make peace and come together. Less communication is necessary.

Performing – This is the stage in which the group begins to really work well. Communication is free flowing.

Network Administrator and Trainer

Network administrators and trainers are two types of support personnel needed primarily when an organization implements a new information system. They perform the following functions:

- **Network administrator:** Network administrators are given access to all areas of the system and must be held to high standards of ethical accountability. These individuals take on the bulk of managing existing systems and planning new systems. They should also help the organization make hardware decisions and manage the lower level information systems employees such as PC specialists and programmers.
- **Trainer:** Trainers teach the organization's staff how to use computer systems. Trainers may be full-time employees of the organization, provided by the software vendor as part of the system contract, or temporary workers. They need to be up to date regarding healthcare information systems and the functions they support.

Analysts, Liaisons, and Programmers

There are three types of **support personnel** that are typically involved in information systems:
- **Analyst:** Analysts must have a background in healthcare information systems. Healthcare information system analysts usually have degrees in the medical field with certificates in computer studies. Their primary job is to define the way in which clinical data is entered into and processed by the information system.
- **Liaison:** Liaisons are hospital employees chosen to work with the information system team while remaining at their primary clinical post. Liaisons act as a conduit between the clinical and information systems staff.
- **Programmers:** Programmers may be full-time hospital employees, but are most likely contract workers or employees of the software vendor. These individuals write the machine language code necessary for system functions. They often work with the analyst and liaison in order to accomplish their tasks.

Security Officer

Since there are many regulatory patient privacy requirements (e.g., HIPAA), **security officers** are essential members of the healthcare information system team. It is important that confidential information is not accessible to unauthorized users or abused by employees. The security officer is responsible for assigning system access codes, making sure passwords are kept secret (and updated), and monitoring the overall use of the system. They may also be in charge of the physical security of the computers and peripherals. A stolen hard drive or laptop computer could contain sensitive information and be a target for information thieves. It is important that the security officer work with the information systems department and the organization's management to create enterprise wide policies and procedures, which describe the proper and ethical use of equipment and information. These standards should apply to all staff members.

Chief Information Officer, Chief Privacy Officer, and Chief e-Health Officer

There are three management level positions that deal with the functioning of an organization's information system:
- **Chief Information Officer:** The chief information officer (CIO) is the head of the information services department. This individual is in charge of hiring information systems staff, budgeting for maintenance of the system, and designing and implementing new systems as needed. Generally, the CIO holds a masters or doctorate degree in computer science.
- **Chief Privacy Officer:** The chief privacy officer (CPO) is a federally mandated position at any facility that treats patients. This individual is responsible for all forms of patient information. The title of CPO is generally bestowed on an employee already working for the organization rather than being an entirely separate job.
- **Chief E-health Officer:** The e-health officer is a relatively new position created by the onset of interactive health websites. The e-health officer is generally in charge of promoting and enabling the use of online interactive patient services.

Compliance Officers, Planning and Recovery Officers, and Interface Engineers

Three information system support roles that are typically held by full-time employees in addition to working under their normal clinical role:

- **Compliance officer:** A compliance officer keeps track of state and federal regulations and accrediting requirements to make sure that the organization is in compliance. This job may be held by someone from the information systems department or by one of the clinical staff members.
- **Planning and recovery officer:** The planning and recovery officer must be sure that disaster plans are up to date and that they are integrated between departments. They must also be aware of what would be required to recover the full functionality of the information system in the event of a disaster.
- **Interface engineer:** The interface engineer should be an employee from the information system department who is capable of making sure that information integrity is maintained when data is exchanged between different systems.

Conflict Resolution

Conflict is an almost inevitable product of teamwork, and the leader must assume responsibility for **conflict resolution.** While conflicts can be disruptive, they can produce positive outcomes by forcing team members to listen to different perspectives and opening dialogue. The team should make a plan for dealing with conflict resolution. The best time for conflict resolution is when differences emerge but before open conflict and hardening of positions occur. The leader must pay close attention to the people and problems involved, listen carefully, and reassure those involved that their points of view are understood. Steps to conflict resolution include:

- Allow both sides to present their side of conflict without bias, maintaining a focus on opinions rather than individuals.
- Encourage cooperation through negotiation and compromise.
- Maintain the focus, providing guidance to keep the discussions on track and avoid arguments.
- Evaluate the need for renegotiation, formal resolution process, or third party.
- Utilize humor and empathy to diffuse escalating tensions.
- Summarize the issues, outlining key arguments.
- Avoid forcing resolution if possible.

System Design Life-Cycle

System Planning

Expert Systems

Expert systems were designed by individuals working in the field of artificial intelligence. These systems are programmed with information that a human expert would use to handle a particular problem, use set rules to analyze the problem, and in some cases provide the user with a list of recommendations. Expert systems are widely used in healthcare to help diagnose and treat patients. The knowledge bases for expert systems are created by a group of individuals who are asked to give guidelines on how they solve very specifically defined problems. Next, the system is created and test cases are used to verify the accuracy of the outcomes. Expert systems may use simple true/false logic or more advanced fuzzy logic. Simple true/false logic design generally asks the user a series of questions to which they answer yes or no. Fuzzy logic attempts to include common uncertainties, but is generally not as accurate as systems designed on true/false logic.

The following is a list of programmed expert systems advantages:
- **Consistency in decision-making.** Given a set input, the returned answer is always the same.
- **A central knowledge depository.** Expert systems can manage a larger database of information than most human experts. Additionally, the knowledge survives staffing changes (e.g., the loss of subject matter experts).
- **Ability to review answers and generate reports.** This allows decision makers unfettered access to information they need at any given time.

The following is a list of programmed expert systems disadvantages:
- **The software lacks "common sense".** It may sometimes provide answers that are not accurate.
- **The logic is "locked down".** The user is unable to deviate from the program in order to be more creative.
- **Programming difficulties.** Programming these types of programs can be difficult due to the need to incorporate high-powered business integrators.
- **Not adaptable.** Once the program has been completed, it is not adaptable to change without major effort.

Elements of a System

There are **six elements** necessary in the **formation of a system**. They are:
- **Interdependency:** There must be multiple components that interact with each other in a concerted way.
- **Inputs:** Data that is placed (input) into the system from an external source (e.g., system users).
- **Process:** The overall functionality that the system contributes its various components towards achieving.

- **Output:** The product of the system. The end result of the various interdependent components of the system. This is usually a distinct product that can only be achieved if the system is operating correctly.
- **Control:** Operation that works to prevent or correct problems as they occur throughout the process. This is usually initiated through a feedback mechanism.
- **Feedback:** An internal control mechanism that allows for the detection and correction of processing problems. This can also include the monitoring of the external environment for an open system.

Open System and Closed System

There are two types of systems: **open** and **closed**. They are defined as follows:
- **Open systems** do not have fixed or permanent boundaries but are instead constantly being re-defined as they interact with the environment. An open system may be a subsystem (e.g., a nurse within a hospital) and can overlap other systems. In computing, an open source program allows access to the source code. This allows customizations and updates from users and programmers in an open environment.
- **Closed systems** are self-contained and isolated from the environment (including other systems). The boundaries of a closed system are distinct and fixed. With the exception of an external energy source, closed systems do not receive input from the environment and all output is contained within the system. A saline IV pump is an example of a closed system. In computing, when the source code is locked (by the vendor) the program acts as a closed system. All adaptations must originate from the vendor.

Network Systems

A **network system** is a group of computers linked together to increase efficiency or distribute computing power. One key reason to use a network system in a healthcare facility is related to data. Patient data must be stored for long periods and accessed by different functional areas within the same facility. By storing patient data in a central server (accessible to all computers connected to the network), the process is made far more efficient and reliable. Another advantage of network systems is that all users share the same software making it easier for the users to share information. In addition, network software licenses are more affordable for the company to purchase. The network software packages are easier to upgrade since only one upgrade to the server is required. Finally, individuals can use the network connection to perform patient consults, proofread each other's work, and send electronic mail (e-mail).

System Development Life Cycle

The system development life cycle is divided up into the following four **phases**:
- **Needs Assessment:** The phase where business requirements are collected from the future users of the system.
- **System Selection:** The phase where an information system is selected that can meet all of the gathered business requirements.
- **Implementation:** The phase in which the system is scaled up and performance tested.
- **Maintenance:** The phase where a help desk is set up (for troubleshooting user problems) and the system is regularly backed-up and updated.

System Selection Process

System selection is an extremely important phase of the system development life cycle. The following are the **three components** of the system selection process:

- **Needs Assessment:** This first action takes place after the decision has been made to purchase a new system or upgrade an existing system. Information is gathered regarding the current state of the art and how the offerings in the marketplace meet the current defined needs of the organization, as well as future needs. Typically, a selection committee attends trade shows and sales meetings that are set up by the potential vendors of the systems.
- **Request for proposal (RFP):** Once the pool of potential vendors has been narrowed down (typically to three), RFPs are sent out. The resulting proposals are then evaluated, references are checked, and the system is evaluated in action (wherever possible).
- **Contract negotiation:** The winning system is then selected and a contract is negotiated with the vendor. Once the contract is approved, implementation plans may proceed.

The following items need to be evaluated when performing the **system selection** portion of the system development life cycle:

- Costs related to the hardware, software and network for the new system.
- Facts about the vendor (e.g., reputation, knowledgeable staff, and financial stability).
- System capabilities in regards to ease of use, user friendly interface, ability to meet the organization's needs, security, expandability, and ability to interface with other systems.

Vendor Attributes

The following is a list of important **attributes** to consider when selecting a **vendor**:

- What is the company's history and financial stability?
- Do they invest in the development of new technologies?
- How many sites currently use the company's systems?
- What other organizations use the system being evaluated?
- What hardware/networking is required for the system architecture?
- Is the company's technology state of the art?
- What other systems and software are compatible with the system?
- What methods of user support are available (phone, internet, etc.) and what is the average response time to a user support request?
- Does the organization have any large upcoming changes for the system to adapt?
- How (and how often) does the company distribute software updates?

Request for Information

Request for information (RFI) is used early in system analysis to gather information from vendors, often in conjunction with requests for proposal and requests for quote. The RFI is often done by letter, although some vendors now use e-mail or accept RFI on websites. The person requesting should outline the type of information needed and give an overview of plans to purchase and install an information system. Many companies have brochures or websites that provide general information about their systems, so sending a list of specific questions may elicit better information. The primary purpose in sending a RFI to a variety of vendors is to help in the elimination and selection process.

Topics for questions may include the following:
- History and financial status of company.
- Lists of current users of company's product and numbers of sites.
- Information about system architecture.
- Hardware and software requirements.
- User support.
- Equipment support/maintenance.
- Ability of equipment to integrate with other systems.

Site Visit

The following information should be gathered when conducting a **site visit**:
- The site's experience regarding the information system's reliability and vendor support services.
- The amount of downtime that has occurred and the primary causes.
- System backup procedures.
- User experiences with the various interfaces to the system.
- Narratives regarding any customizations to the system.
- A log of the amount of hours of training that were required.
- System security performance.
- Overall satisfaction with the system.

Request for Proposal

The following information should be included in a **request for proposal** (RFP):
- A description of the organization.
- The organization's mission statement, goals, and objectives.
- The organizational structure.
- The type of healthcare facility.
- The proportion of clients in each pay type.
- The patient and facility statistics.
- The overall system requirements.
- The criteria for evaluating responses to the RFP.
- The deadline for submission of the requested information.

Steering Committee

The following are the overall **steps** in the **formation of a steering committee**:
- **Step 1:** Form a steering committee to evaluate the current information system and begin the research process for the new system.
- **Step 2:** Staff the steering committee with representatives from all levels of the organization that will use the new system.
- **Step 3:** Establish a leader of the steering committee that will own the process and report progress.
- **Step 4:** Establish the steering committee's goals and objectives.
- **Step 5:** Determine if an experienced outside consultant is needed to handle complex technical issues, and/or save time.

The following **tasks** should be carried out by the **steering committee** when researching a new information system:

- Verify that the project fits into the organization's goals and objectives as stated in the mission statement.
- Reach a consensus on the business requirements that the new information system needs to satisfy.
- Scan the internal environment within the organization to assess where the current information system is not adequate.
- Look to the future to assess the longevity of the new system and how it can evolve to meet the organization's needs for the next three to five years.

Strategic Planning

Applying the System Theory to the Strategic Planning Process

Systems take in information (called inputs), process it, and then produce new information (called outputs). Feedback controls the processes that occur within a system. The functional parts of a system and its processes are interdependent. A change or problem in one part of a system can affect the system's overall processes and this may cause problems for other parts of the system down the line. A secondary malfunction is defined as a change in one part of a system due to a problem in another part of the system. Problems must therefore be corrected at the area of the primary malfunction in order to prevent a secondary malfunction. If a problem affects the system's functions, it can also affect the output. To simplify **systems theory**, a system is more than the sum of its parts and is not equal to the function of its individual parts.

Strategic Planning

Enterprise-wide strategic planning requires that an organization look at needs of the organization, community, and customers and establish both short-term (2-4 years) and long-term (10-15 years) goals. Strategic planning must be based on internal and external assessments to determine the present course of action, needed changes, priorities, and methodologies to effect change. The focus of strategic planning must be on the development of services based on identified customer needs and then the marketing of those services. Enterprise-wide strategic planning includes:
- Collecting data and doing an external analysis of customer needs.
- Analyzing internal services and functions.
- Identifying and understanding key issues, including the strengths and weaknesses of the organization, potential opportunities, and negative impacts.
- Developing revised mission and vision statements that identify core values.
- Establishing specific goals and objectives.

The following **major steps** are used in strategic planning:
- Develop a mission statement.
- Determine goals and objectives.
- Create a strategic plan to achieve the goals and objectives that includes:
  - Identify potential solutions.
  - Select a course of action.
  - Implement the chosen solution.
  - Conduct regular evaluations including feedback from those involved in the strategic plan.

The following common **goals** are relevant to **strategic planning** in healthcare information systems:
- Computer systems designed to support business and clinical decisions.
- Stay abreast of current technology.
- Using the organization's technological innovations as a marketing tool.
- To meet regulatory requirements.
- To aid efficiency and overall productivity.
- To improve the accuracy and dependability of patient data (especially tracking).

The following **questions** should be asked when performing **strategic planning** for information systems:

- Is the core operating system open or closed? Can programmers access the program's actual code?
- What technology is the system built upon?
- What is the user interface? Is it user friendly?
- Does the system comply with required standards (such as HL7)?
- How easy is it to access raw data and create reports?
- How is the system performance measured?
- Can users customize their views?
- How many users can access the system simultaneously?
- Is the system upgradeable?
- Will the system reduce or eliminate paper?
- What is the timeline for implementation?

Both the external and internal **environments** should be examined when performing **strategic planning**. In terms of the external environment, the major item of interest would be the state of technology. Some questions to ask include:

- Has the hardware and/or software been updated by the suppliers?
- Do we as an organization need to move up to the new level?
- What are our competitors or peers up to?
- Would an update in technology become a competitive advantage?

In terms of internal environment, this information should be readily available through feedback from the users of the current informatics systems. In addition, any changes in business processes that require new capabilities should also be examined.

Information Needs Assessment

Needs Assessment

The following items need to be evaluated when performing the **needs assessment** portion of the system development life cycle:
- Compatibility and connectivity of the hardware and software that will be incorporated into the system.
- Amount of downtime required for system testing and installation.
- Set up of the test and live environments.
- System response time and number of concurrent users.
- User support system.
- Administration of the system.
- Security parameters of the system.
- Disaster recovery contingency plans.
- User interface and ability to retrieve reports.
- System routines used for business processes such as hospital registration, records, and billing.

Organizational Goals

Organizational goals are set based upon a needs assessment. The first step is for management to agree on the upcoming needs of the organization. These needs may be long-term, short-term, or a combination of both. Once the needs have been determined, performance goals for individuals and teams should be set to meet the organization's needs. It is important that the individual goals are specific, measurable, and time based. The goals should be distributed across the organization to align efforts in meeting the core needs. Regular milestones should also be set to assure that progress is being made.

Gap Analysis

Gap analysis is a method used to determine the steps required to move from a current state or actual performance or situation to a new one or potential performance or situation and the "gap" between the two that requires action or resources. Essentially gap analysis answers the questions "What is our current situation?" and "What do we want it to become?" Gap analysis includes the determination of the resources and time required to achieve the target goal. Steps to gap analysis include:
- Assessing the current situation and listing important factors, such as performance levels, costs, staffing, and satisfaction, and all processes.
- Identifying the current outcomes of the processes in place.
- Identifying the target outcomes for projected processes.
- Outlining the process required to achieve target outcomes.
- Identifying the gaps that are present between the current process and goal.
- Identifying resources and methods to close the gaps.

Resource Use

Resource use refers to the consideration of all factors related to the planning and delivery of quality products and activities. Resources may be allotted to the physical environment for building or remodeling, staffing, equipment, literature, training, and outreach programs. Use review requires consideration of individual safety, program effectiveness, and cost. Interventions should be safe, effective, and affordable for each individual. Decisions should take into consideration rising health care costs and how to maximize the use of resources while continuing to provide quality professional development activities. The goal of resource use is to provide quality, cost-effective programs while using the best-qualified staff and appropriate resources.

Inventory

Inventory describes the amount of material or equipment on hand, which should be reviewed at least once a year. In many cases, reordering is done when the amount of a particular item drops to a certain pre-established level. Just-in-time ordering is done when stock is almost depleted. Automatic reordering of supplies is easy when inventories are computerized. In some cases, departments have open accounts that can be used for small purchases without bidding. For large purchases (especially in public institutions), the nurse should state exactly (i.e., include brand names when appropriate) which items are to be purchased on a bid form. The bids are then sent to prospective bidders (at least three) in a competitive bid process. Organizations vary in what bids are acceptable. Some only accept the lowest bid, while others accept the best bid (e.g., those supplying brand names rather than substituting with generics). Many organizations have private purchase plans that allow them to purchase directly without bids or lease equipment, which is less expensive initially.

Staffing Management

Staffing management involves both clinical staff (e.g., nurses) and nonclinical staff (e.g., housekeeping staff, office personnel). Important issues include the following:
- Workforce size and distribution, including full-time equivalent staff members, needed.
- Educational resources, such as training programs, and availability of trained personnel, including professional staff and support staff.
- Staff training, ongoing need for staff development, and opportunities for certification or advancement.
- Demographics (e.g., age, economic levels, ethnic backgrounds, lifestyles).
- Incentives for career advancement, including increases in income, promotion, and certification.
- Staff turnover, burnout, and an ongoing need for recruitment.
- Organizational structure.
- Financial resources available.
- Cost-effective staffing and billable provision of care.
- Reimbursement (e.g., Medicare, Medicaid, health insurance, private pay).
- Supervision/feedback.
- Organization-wide strategies for staffing.

Cost-Benefit Analysis

A **cost-benefit analysis** considers the cost that results from an undesirable event taking place and compares it to the cost of an intervention to prevent that event to demonstrate potential savings. Consider the following example:

- Computer repair overtime costs related to improper computer use are $125/hour. If the institution averages 10 hours of overtime a month due to this problem, then the annual cost would be:

$$10 \times \$125 \times 12 = \$15,000$$

- If the intervention to remedy this problem included staff training materials ($400), instructor costs ($2000), and compliance monitoring costs ($1500), then the total intervention cost would be:

$$\$400 + \$2000 + \$1500 = \$3900$$

- If the intervention were to decrease overtime costs by 80% to 2 overtime hours a month, then the annual savings would be:

$$80\% \times \$15,000 = \$12,000$$

- Subtracting the intervention costs from the savings gives the annual cost-benefit:

$$\$12,000 - \$3900 = \$8100$$

Cost-Effective Analysis, Efficacy Studies, and Incremental Cost-Effectiveness Ratio

A **cost-effective analysis** measures the effectiveness of an intervention in terms of the monetary savings. For example, each year, about 2 million nosocomial infections result in 90,000 deaths and an estimated $6.7 billion in additional health costs. From that perspective, decreasing infections should reduce costs, but there are human savings in suffering as well, on which it is difficult to place a dollar value. If a hospital sustains 200 nosocomial infections per year, and the average infection adds 12 days to hospitalization, then the results a 20% reduction in nosocomial infections would be calculated as follows:

$$20\% \times 200 = 40; 40 \times 12 = 480.$$

A 20% reduction in infections cuts 480 patient hospitalization days.

Efficacy studies may compare a series of cost-benefit analyses to determine the intervention with the best cost-benefit. They may also be used for process or product evaluation. For example, a study might be done to determine the effective use of four different types of computers to determine which type resulted in the fewest errors that resulted in added costs, thus saving the most money. **Incremental cost-effectiveness ratio** is the ratio of cost change to outcome change.

Cost-Utility Analysis

Cost-utility analysis (CUA) is a subtype of cost-effective analysis; however, the results are more difficult to quantify and use to justify expense because a CUA measures the benefit to society (e.g., decreasing teen pregnancy). Often the standards used to quantify a CUA are somewhat subjective. A CUA compares a variety of outcomes (e.g., increased life expectancy, decreased suffering) in relation to the quality-adjusted-life-year. A scale is used with 1 being normal health and 0 being death. A health condition is assigned a number on this scale, which is referred to as its "utility."

When calculating outcomes with a CUA, an intervention is evaluated on whether or not it increases the utility score and thereby increases life expectancy or improves life circumstances by x number of years. Thus, the results of this type of analysis are not expressed as monetary values but rather societal values.

Return on Investment and Payback Period

Return on investment (ROI) refers to an accounting calculation that is used to determine the value that an investment provides. Consider the following example ROI calculation for buying a new $20,000 piece of equipment for an employee. In addition to the cost of the investment, three other quantities must be known:

- The annual cost of the employee who will use the equipment; example: $80,000
- The percentage of work time that the employee will use the equipment; example: 25%
- The estimated (or calculated, if the analysis is done after the purchase) percentage increase in efficiency over the prior system; example: 30%

Multiplying these three values gives the cost savings resulting from the purchase:
$$\$80,000 \times 0.25 \times 0.30 = \$6000$$

ROI is then expressed as the savings divided by the cost:
$$ROI = \frac{\$6000}{\$20,000} = 30\%$$

The **payback period (PBP)** for an investment refers to the amount of time required for the savings resulting from the investment to equal the cost of the investment. To calculate payback period, divide the cost of the investment by the savings it provides:
$$PBP = \frac{\$20,000}{\$6000} = 3.33 \text{ years or 40 months}$$

The payback period is essentially the inverse of the ROI. because you are dividing the cost of the investment by the savings to determine the number of years until the investment has paid for itself.

Internal Customer–Supplier Relationships

Internal customer-supplier relationships in an organization must be identified and understood. Internal customers are those directly involved in product or health care delivery, such as those on the Board of Directors, clerical staff, administrative personnel, nursing personnel, medical support staff, physicians, human resources personnel, plant managers, pharmacists, and volunteer staff. A customer is, by definition, a receiver. Internal customers need others in the work environment to provide some type of product or service so that they may function, and they, in turn, provide a product or service to others, so each internal customer is also a supplier. Vertical customer–supplier relationships, such as between administration and nursing staff, are sometimes more obvious than the equally important horizontal relationships, such as between floor nurses, which can involve cooperative measures to ensure that quality care is provided. Identifying customer–supplier relationships should be part of strategic planning to increase internal awareness and improve methods of meeting the various customers' needs.

External Customer–Supplier Relationships

External customer-supplier relationships are critical to an organization because these customers receive products or services supplied by the organization. External customers include patients and their families, private physicians, vendors, insurance companies, government regulatory agencies, lawyers, and others in the community. As with internal customers, each external customer is both a receiver of products or goods and a supplier. For example, a regulatory agency provides regulations and guidelines as a supplier and then receives reports in return as a customer. This symbiotic relationship must be clearly understood because the external customer–supplier relationship is one over which the organization often has less direct control, so identification of the customers' needs through surveys, interviews, focus groups, research, and brainstorming can help to clarify and improve these relationships.

Planning Education

Over-the-Shoulder Instruction

Over-the-shoulder instruction is a learner-centered strategy in which the instructor moves about the classroom monitoring the learner's progress rather than standing at the front of the classroom and lecturing or providing instructor-focused teaching. Most instruction is computerized learning, so student attention is often focused on technology. Advantages are that this strategy allows for one-on-one instruction with individual learners as the instructor observes a need or the learner requests assistance, and the instructor is better able to monitor individual progress. However, disadvantages are that many learners may have the same questions so the instructor may waste time answering the same questions multiple times to individual students. Additionally, if the group of learners is large, the instructor may not be able to address the needs or questions of all students. In some cases, the learning environment may seem impersonal because of less interaction with the instructor.

One-on-One Instruction vs. Group Instruction

Both **one-on-one instruction** and **group instruction** have a place in patient/family education.
- **One-on-one instruction** is the most costly for an institution because it is time intensive. However, it allows more interaction with the instructor and allows learners to have more control over the process by asking questions or having the instructor repeat explanations or demonstrations. One-on-one instruction is especially valuable when learners must master particular skills or if confidentiality is important.
- **Group instruction** is less costly because the needs of a number of people can be met at one time. Group presentations are more planned and usually scheduled for a particular time period (e.g., an hour), so learners have less control. Questioning is usually limited and usually only at the end of a session. Group instruction allows learners with similar needs to interact. Group instruction is especially useful for general types of instruction, such as managing diet or other lifestyle issues.

Just-in-Time Presentations

Just-in-time presentations are used when learners need to use the information immediately. For example, if teaching learners to access data in a new computerized system, a supportive overview of the system and its purpose may be given right before hands-on practice and basic instruction about use. However, only when the learners need to access data is the presentation about data access provided. This allows learners to draw on what they have learned immediately without the typical memory loss that occurs when people try to retrieve information they learned at an earlier time. Just-in-time presentations are especially useful with procedural information that is not very complex and that helps people master a specific task. A training session may include both supportive information given immediately before practice and just-in-time presentations interspersed throughout the session.

Problem-Based Learning

Problem-based learning was developed by McMaster University in the 1960s. It is learner-centered with the instructor serving as facilitator rather than lecturer. The learners are presented with a problem and must search for the solution. Problem-based learning focuses on promoting the learners' ability to use critical thinking and problem-solving skills, increasing motivation. This process of problem-solving is believed to enhance transfer so that information learned in one context is internalized and can be used in other contexts as well. While effective, this method requires more preparation time and may require an extended learning period while the learners identify the problem and attempt to formulate a solution. The teacher/facilitator can guide the learners by helping them to ask questions that lead to solutions.

Teaching Models

Audiovisual tutorials: These are very effective for supplementary material and independent study.

Independent study: This is geared toward the needs of the individual who can self-pace; materials may be internet-based or paper-based and may include audiovisual materials.

Goal-focused: Learners are presented with a goal, and all materials and activities are aimed at achieving that goal.

Guided focus: Learning takes place outside a formal classroom with materials provided or recommended by the instructor.

Anchored: Activities are based on problem-solving in relation to realistic case studies.

Collaborative: Learners work together to complete a learning activity.

Project-based: Learners develop materials (e.g., videos, website, pamphlets) regarding a topic.

Problem-based: Learners work in teams to solve problems.

Cognitive apprenticeship: Instructors model, and learners analyze and apply processes.

Simulations: Learners actively participate in simulated activities.

Direct instruction: This is an instructor-focused presentation.

Cooperative: Small teams work together through a variety of activities to master a subject, with each member responsible for self-learning and learning from others on the team.

Blended/Hybrid Learning

Blended/hybrid learning encompasses a wide range of teaching methodologies. Blended/hybrid learning combines traditional lecture-type, instructor-focused delivery with more modern approaches, such as computer-based instruction. With blended/hybrid learning, the instructor often balances classroom learning with out-of-classroom learning, using various technologies, such as smart phones, IPods, and IPads to access internet-based, computerized modules or applications. When designing a blended/hybrid course, the instructor must consider the expected outcomes and competencies the learners must master, the size and nature of the audience, the location of learners or classrooms, and the available resources. A typical blended/hybrid class begins with an introduction by the instructor and then moves to other formats, such as computer-based learning, while the instructor assumes the role of facilitator, using just-in-time presentations and combining over-the-shoulder, one-on-one, and group instruction as necessary to meet the class goals.

Selection of Teaching Materials and Resources

It is impractical to believe that the nurse can produce all **teaching materials** and **resources**, but careful consideration must be given to the **selection** process.

- **Price** ranges from free to hundreds or even thousands of dollars for educational materials, which may be handouts, videos, posters, or entire courses or series of courses available online. The nurse must first consider the budget and then look for material within those monetary constraints. Government agencies, such as the Centers for Disease Control, often have posters and handouts as well as PowerPoint presentations and videos available for download online at no cost.
- **Quality** varies considerably as well. The nurse should consider the goal and objectives before choosing materials, and the materials should be evaluated to determine if they cover all needed information in a clear and engaging manner.
- **Currency** must be considered as well. If material will soon be outdated because of changes in regulations, then it will have to be replaced.

Written Handouts and Paper Materials

Written handouts or other **paper materials** are a fixture in classes, but many end up in the wastebasket without ever being used; thus, thought should be given to what useful information should be in the handouts:

- Handouts that simply copy a PowerPoint presentation or repeat everything in the presentation are less helpful than those that summarize the main points.
- Giving out handouts immediately before a discussion ensures that most of the class will be looking at the handout instead of the speaker. Thus, handouts should be placed in a folder or binder and passed out before the class meets so students can peruse them in advance; for example, handouts can be passed out at the end of class in preparation for the next class.
- Handouts can be used to provide guidance or worksheets for small-group discussions.
- Posters (with drawings or pictures) that can be placed on bulletin boards are useful.
- Handouts should be easily readable and not smudged copies of newspaper articles or small print text.

Electronic and Audiovisual Materials

There are a number of issues that must be considered when teaching a course and determining the appropriate audiovisual and handout materials. The physical environment is a major consideration, especially when using **electronic** and **audiovisual materials**.

- First, everyone in the room must be able to hear and see. In a small room, a television or computer screen may suffice, but in a large space, a projection screen must be used.
- Another issue is lighting. Some projectors have low resolution and the lights need to be turned off, dimmed, or windows covered. Turning lights on and off a dozen times during a presentation can be very distracting. A small portable light at a speaker podium or an alternate presentation can be used.
- Text size for presentations is another issue: PowerPoint or other presentations that include text must be of a sufficient font size to be read from the back of the room.

Videos, Videoconferencing, and Teleconferencing

Videos are a useful adjunct to teaching as they reduce the time needed for one-on-one instruction (increasing cost-effectiveness). Good-quality videos can be expensive to produce, although commercial products are available. Passive presentation of videos, such as in a waiting area, has limited value, but focused viewing in which the educator discusses the purpose of the video presentation before viewing and then is available for discussion after viewing can be very effective. Videos are also effective tools for demonstrating patient care techniques, such as wound care. Additionally, videos can be placed on course or learning management systems for anytime access. Providing focused questions for use during the video presentation helps increase retention by keeping active involvement. **Videoconferencing** and **teleconferencing** allow for audiovisual collaboration at a distance and can be a valuable tool for education, providing access to experts without the transportation costs. In teleconferencing, students may be at multiple sites while interacting with each other and an instructor.

Hospital Information System

The **hospital information system (HIS)** can provide real practice for students and trainees using hardware and software programs that they will need when caring for patients. Nursing students can use HIS to generate care plans and do mapping rather than doing this in the traditional time-consuming paper method. The students and trainees should be able to access fictitious patient files and retrieve and enter information, but security must be in place to prevent access to actual patient files for training purposes as this violates the Health Insurance Portability and Accountability Act (HIPAA) regulations. Additionally, existing staff, such as nurse managers, should be taught how to access data from patient census records and electronic health records (EHRs) to plan staffing, organize care, and promote patient safety. Any training involving HIS and EHR must review HIPAA regulations as well as methods to ensure data security and patient confidentiality.

Classroom Response Systems

Electronic **classroom response systems (CRS)** include the use of clickers to respond to questions or educational content. For example, if an instructor asks the class a question, all students can answer with the clicker, which beams responses wirelessly to a computer, so the instructor can immediately determine if the students understood the question and responded appropriately. This is especially valuable in large groups where quiet students (or those in the back) may have little input into discussions. Additionally, responses can be projected from the computer onto a screen and, in some cases, graphed, so that students are able to see the results of the questions visually. One major advantage to the clicker is that those who might be afraid to answer or unsure can do so privately. Students using clickers often remain more actively engaged in the learning process.

Help Tools

A variety of **help tools** are available for education, including the following:
- **Learning aids:** Questions, guides, maps, pictures, charts, illustrations, outlines, or diagrams can be used to support lecture or computer-based training.
- **Internet tools:** These can include websites that provide specific educational content and information updates, such as the Skin Care Network at NursingCenter.com (Lippincott), and interactive websites. Additionally, chat tools and message boards may provide valuable support for students.

- **Software applications:** Software is available for training on almost every health care topic and usually includes interactivity and audiovisual presentations. Many applications are available for portable devices as well.
- **Books:** Many books are now available in electronic versions, making access less expensive and more easily transported.
- **Multimedia:** Compact discs, DVDs, and streaming videos combine sound and images with hardware/software to deliver educational content.

Areas of Training for Information Systems

Training employees on a new computer system should take the user through each part of the system that they will be working with. They should be introduced to the exact steps needed to perform each function that is required by their job. Simulations of potential challenging situations should be practiced. Additional features such as basic troubleshooting help screens and online tutorials should also be introduced to the trainees. Specific **areas for training staff** on information systems include:
- The basics of how the computer system works. This includes both the hardware and software.
- How the system impacts their areas of responsibility. This should include some "hands on" training at the individuals' workstation.
- The computer support resources should be painstakingly outlined so that the staff member knows exactly what is available to them and at what times.

End-Users and Informatics Staff

Developing informatics competencies among **end-users** and **informatics staff** requires intensive and comprehensive training and institutional support. A variety of different training procedures, such as one-on-one or instructor-led classrooms, may be used. Training should include the following:
- Policies regarding computers, including privacy issues, penalties, and failure to comply with policies
- Access policies and issues regarding misuse (e.g., viewing nonauthorized materials)
- Preimplementation steps to prepare end-users for changes and to inform and educate informatics staff
- Basic computer literacy information
- Workflow diagrams outlining changes occurring with transition from manual to automatic systems
- Scenarios with step-by-step instructions
- Access and use of help documents and online tutorials
- Generation of error messages, including avoidance and error correction
- Causes of screen & system freezing and troubleshooting methods
- Elements specific to the organization's system
- Maintenance and troubleshooting for hardware and software
- Methods of information retrieval
- Managing downtimes (both scheduled and nonscheduled) and backup systems

Information System-Training Plan

An **information system training** plan should include the following elements:
- A training mission statement to demonstrate the organization's commitment to the training process.
- A needs assessment (who will be trained, what will be taught, what resources are necessary, how much time will be spent, and where training will occur).
- The training modes that will be used: self-paced, on-the-job, or instructor led.
- Whether the trainers are in-house staff or contractors.
- The amount of time needed before the staff is deemed competent.
- The amount of money that will be spent on training.
- The methods that will be used to determine training effectiveness.

Choosing a Training Site

The following is a list of factors to consider when choosing a **site** for information system training:
- Is there space available to conduct the training on-site or will an off-site facility be needed?
- Is the training budget adequate to allow for the option of off-site training?
- Are their enough computer terminals for all of the trainees or will they have to share a terminal?
- Is the site properly configured with power outlets and network connections?
- If the training is at an off-site location, is it convenient to the trainees in terms of parking and proximity to work?
- Is the site prepared with all of the required training materials?

Choosing an Information System Trainer

The following characteristics should be taken into account when **selecting a trainer** for information systems:
- **Experience**: Has the trainer worked with hospital information systems (HIS) previously? How knowledgeable are they regarding the newly installed system?
- **Style**: How does the trainer work in group situations? Are they good at the communication and coaching aspects of the training session?
- **Organizational fit:** Is the individual familiar with the training approach and philosophy that the organization prefers?
- **Working with upper management**: Will the individual be able to train users on the specialized departmental level?

Scheduling User-Training Sessions

It can be challenging to train the staff of an organization that runs 24 hours a day, 7 days a week (such as a hospital). Finding the best **time to train staff** members will depend on their overall availability. People may often have to come in late (and be too tired to concentrate) if they are scheduled for a training session after their shift ends. The best strategy may be to allow individuals an entire day for training purposes. It may also be necessary to offer training during all three shifts (i.e., 24 hours a day) in order to accommodate shift personnel. Trainees should be given materials to review in advance of the training session so that they will be fully prepared. Training should also be timed to occur as close to the go-live date as possible so that the new information will be remembered.

Assessing Ongoing Training Needs

Although extensive training should be completed before implementation of an information system, **ongoing training needs** must be assessed and training instituted. Methods of assessing needs include the following:

- **End-user questionnaires and interviews:** Determine perceptions of need and user acceptance/attitudes. Staff members often know where their training needs lie and appreciate input.
- **Real-time observations:** Note efficiency of use, correct or incorrect use, and time needed to carry out activities to note where changes would improve functioning.
- **Analysis of errors/repairs:** Note patterns of errors (e.g., frequency, time, units), such as increased input errors in a single department, which suggest the need for more targeted training. This type of analysis may be the most cost-effective as it trains only those who need improved skills.
- **Reviewing staff changes:** Note new additions to staff because they may have no or little or no training in use of the system.

Training Materials and Proficiency Testing

Choosing the appropriate **materials** (both those supplied by the vendor and supplementary) for information system training is a key aspect of the learning process. The materials should reflect and support the operation of the live information system. The materials should be clear, concise, and targeted at the comprehension level of the trainees. In addition to the training materials, job aids should be available at the trainee workstation. These job aids should be step-by-step instructions as to how to work with the new system. In addition, of critical importance in training is **proficiency testing**. The degree to which the trainees have absorbed the knowledge should be evaluated. There are two types of proficiency examinations: criterion referenced or norm referenced. Criterion referenced measures assess each test taker against a set correct value (this measure is the most commonly used). Norm referenced exams grade individuals directly against one another.

Choosing a Training Method for a New Information System

The following four factors should be considered when choosing a **training method** for a new information system:

- **Time:** Different training methods take various amounts of time to prepare and perform (e.g., in-person or self-taught)
- **Cost:** This includes the cost of trainers, equipment, and the number of hours that employees will need to spend away from their job.
- **Learning styles:** It is important to consider the predominant successful training style for the organization (what works best for the majority of trainees). This may be determined by the demographics (age, gender, education) of the trainee pool.
- **Learning retention:** Retention of training concepts may be much higher if the training is "hands-on" (or in-person) rather that self-taught.

Multimedia and Tutorial Methods of Online Training

Online multimedia advantages:
- Interactive: The trainee can access live feedback.
- Improves retention: Instructor may be asked questions.
- Tests of proficiency can be used: Real-time evaluations may be conducted with the trainees.

Online multimedia disadvantages:
- Instructor and trainees must be available at predefined times.
- Technology related problems may cancel the session.
- Trainees need access to a computer and network connection.

Online tutorials advantages:
- The tutorial is available to the trainees 24 hours a day (7 days a week).
- The trainee can revisit the sections they are having trouble with or need additional time.
- Off-line examinations can be administered.

Online tutorials disadvantages:
- The success of a tutorial is dependent on the richness and functionality of the design.
- The trainee may not be as focused on the materials as they would be in a live setting.

E-Mail and Video Methods of Training

The following advantages and disadvantages of the **e-mail and video methods** of training include:

Email advantages
- Trainees receive training materials electronically.
- E-mail messages are easy to assemble and send to targeted trainees.

Email disadvantages
- Trainees must open the mail and follow the instructions for completing.
- Reponses might be slow or non-existent without stringent follow-up procedures.

Video advantages
- Videos are available 24 hours a day, 7 days a week.
- Exposes many trainees to a single point of training material.
- Easy to distribute and can be shared by trainees within uniform functional areas.

Video disadvantages
- Requires expensive cameras and production techniques.
- The instructor must be familiar with presenting the training material through the video medium.

Computer Based Training (CBT) for Information Systems

Computer Based Training (CBT) is a more popular and efficient type of training for information systems. Advantages and disadvantages of computer-based training include:

Advantages

- Self-paced: The trainee can go through the materials as fast (or slow) as they choose.
- Interactive: There is instant feedback regarding correct/incorrect responses to exercises.
- Availability: The training is available per the trainee's schedule.
- Modules: The training can be broken up into easily completed modules.

Disadvantages

- Construction: It takes a lot of time and labor to develop and maintain a good CBT system.
- Lack of coaching: Trainees must learn without the help of knowledgeable coaches.

Instructor Led Classes for Training

Instructor led training is one of the most popular types of training for information systems.

The **advantages** of instructor led training are:
- Uniformity: All trainees are exposed to the same material at the same time.
- Coaching: Trainer is able to interact one on one with trainees.
- Question and answer period: Trainees can have their questions answered immediately.
- Demonstrations: The instructor can demonstrate the use of the test information system (set up for the class).
- Tests of proficiency can be used.

The **disadvantages** of instructor led training are:
- The effectiveness of the training depends on the quality and knowledge base of the trainer.
- Larger class sizes can make training experience less effective.
- The trainer must keep the level of training in line with the average trainee's experience.

Internet-Based and On-the-Job Training Approaches

Internet Based Training: Internet-based training delivers content directly to students via the internet.
- **Advantages**: Accessible from any PC that is connected to the network, Available 24 hours a day
- **Disadvantages**: Highly trained webmaster needed, Intranet must already be in place
- **Tips**: Online learner assessment is included.

On-the-Job Training: On-the-job training is delivered to the student in-person usually at the work site itself.
- **Advantages**: Can be tailored to the individual, Learning is applied immediately, Proficiency is tested by the trainer
- **Disadvantages**: Productivity is less during training time, Bad habits can easily be passed on, Interruptions are extremely bothersome
- **Tips**: Trainer should be knowledgeable in adult education, Works well for lower level staff

Support Personnel Who Work with Healthcare Information Systems

All healthcare information systems have a variety of support personnel. These are the people who work to keep the system updated and running well:

- **Super User:** A super user is an employee who has some advanced knowledge about computers (and computer systems) and is familiar with the work done at the department level. A hospital may have a super user in each unit or department.
- **Help Desk Personnel:** These are the people who answer user questions over the phone or in response to e-mail. If the problem is too difficult to work out over the phone, they may send someone to the user's location. A hospital must have a 24-hour information system help line for the users.
- **PC Specialist:** A PC specialist usually has a bachelor's degree in computer science and assists with training and system setup (including upgrades). They may also install software on individual devices (e.g., Pocket PC).

Super User and Job-Aid Training Approaches

There are two major on-the-job training methods for conducting information system training:

Super user: The super user is a regular user of the system who has in-depth knowledge of the information system.

- **Advantages** - Understands the clinical areas and the information system
  Any user may apply for this position
- **Disadvantages** - Must take time away from clinical position
  Must attend information system meetings
- **Tips** - Is a good assistant trainer; Can help other users on the job

Job aids: Job aids are learning tools used at the workstation.

- **Advantages** - Lessens the need to memorize large amounts of information
  Lessens the amount of time needed for dedicated training
- **Disadvantages** - Access must be complete
  Aids must be up to date
- **Tips** - User friendliness is key
  All users must be given same information

Peer Training and Self-Directed Text-Based Courses

There are two basic methods for carrying out information system training:

Peer Training: This is a method in which new users of the system are trained by existing users (their peers). The new employee shadows the peer and is coached on the proper operation of the system.

- **Advantages** - Training is tailored directly to the function needed
  Proficiency can be easily tested
- **Disadvantages** - Trainer may not be knowledgeable in principles of education
  Existing bad habits can be easily passed on
- **Tips** - Trainer should be knowledgeable in adult education
  Works well for lower level staff

Self-Directed Text-Based Courses: This method is based on self-directed (and self-paced) training by use of the provided materials. The materials are usually in the form of workbooks that can be studied at home or during breaks on the job. There is very little interaction with the subject matter experts.

- **Advantages** - Individual works at their own pace
  Proficiency is easily tested
  Hospital system does not need to be in place for training to go on
- **Disadvantages** - Personal motivation has to be high
- **Tips** - Materials must be highly structured

Training Process for Naive Computer Users

For employees that have little or no computer experience, remedial **training** is required. These individuals may feel intimidated by the idea of working with a computer system for the first time. It is important to address their fears and make them feel comfortable in the training environment. It may be useful to introduce them to basic computer use with a game (or other skill building software) before moving on to something more complex. These individuals may need to be taught basic computer skills (e.g., how to use a mouse and how to print documents).

Disaster Recovery

Disaster recovery procedures should be taught to users in the event the system "crashes" or goes down for a period of time. It is important to have a back up plan because all information systems are subject to service failures (e.g., power outages or networking problems). The backup procedures should allow the users to continue to perform their assigned tasks in another independent manner (such as paper-based) while the system is down. During training, users should be taken through the backup procedures for the entire organization and for their own department or unit. Additionally, the users should be taught how to backfill the data that was captured while the system was down (once it comes back up).

Troubleshooting of System Problems

Basic **troubleshooting** should be taught to all users of the system. This would include re-boot procedures (for a frozen screen), changing passwords, how to properly edit data entries, and when to contact the support desk. Because every system is unique, users must learn the proper procedures to follow when problems arise. Also, learning when to report system performance (i.e., when the system is running slow or oddly) to the system administrator may help avoid a much larger problem.

Instructing and Advising Staff on Changes in Policies, Procedures, or Working Standards

Changes in policies, **procedures**, or **working standards** are common, and the quality professional is responsible for educating the staff about changes related to processes, which should be communicated in an effective and timely manner.

- **Policies** are usually changed after a period of discussion and review by administration and staff, so all staff should be made aware of policies under discussion. Preliminary information should be disseminated to staff regarding the issue during meetings or through printed notices.
- **Procedures** may be changed to increase efficiency or improve patient safety often as the result of surveillance and outcome data. Procedural changes are best communicated in workshops with demonstrations. Posters and handouts should be available as well.
- **Working standards** are often changed because of regulatory or accrediting requirements; this information should be covered extensively in a variety of ways: discussions, workshops, and handouts so that the implications are clearly understood.

Clinical Work Flow Analysis

Clinical Flow Chart

A **clinical flow chart** is a schematic representation of a process and is often used to analyze quality improvement, particularly when looking for solutions to a problem. Typically, the following symbols are used:

- **Parallelogram:** input and output (start/end).
- **Arrow:** direction of flow.
- **Diamond:** conditional decision (yes/no or true/false).
- **Circle:** connectors with diverging paths with multiple arrows coming in but only one going out.

A variety of other symbols may be used to indicate different functions. Flow goes from top to bottom and left to right. Flow charts help people visualize how a process is carried out and to examine a process for problems. Flow charts may also be used to plan a process before it is used. Flow charts may demonstrate critical pathways to outline treatment options or paths related to findings.

Storyboard

A **storyboard** is a visual representation of the actions of a team, including data analysis and decisions, during the performance improvement process. It is usually done on a firm poster board and may be 3–4 feet square. It is somewhat like a giant flow chart with arrows or lines connecting one piece of information to the next. The storyboard may be used to present summary reports and is also a tool used in continuous quality improvement. The storyboard may include a variety of items or information, such as the following:

- Charts
- Diagrams
- Pictures
- Text
- Illustrations
- Statistics

Because the storyboard is meant to provide easy access to information about team activities, text is usually minimal.

Gantt Chart

A **Gantt chart** is used for developing improvement projects to manage schedules and estimate time needed to complete tasks. It is a bar chart with a horizontal time scale that presents a visual representation of the beginning and end points of time when different steps in a process should be completed. Gantt charts are a component of project management software programs. The Gantt chart is usually created after initial brainstorming and creation of a time line and action plans. Steps to create a Gantt chart include the following:

1. List the name of the process at the top.
2. Create a chart with a timeline of days, weeks, or months (as appropriate for process) horizontally across the top.
3. List tasks vertically on the left of the chart.

Draw horizontal lines or bars from the expected beginning point to the expected end point for each task. These may be color-coded to indicate which individual or team is responsible for completing the task.

Data-Flow Diagrams

Data-flow diagrams show how data flow into a system and from one process to another, presenting a graphic representation of a system and its processes. The diagram is a simplified flow chart that uses only four symbols, which are labeled during diagramming:

- **Square:** external entity or sources of data or external destinations. An entity is named.
- **Rounded rectangle:** process in inputting and outputting data. This is named with verb and object (but does not include word "process," and there is no subject). Data flow is from left to right and top to bottom. Each rounded rectangle represents only one process (so "and" is not used).
- **Arrow (line with arrowhead):** direction of data flow. Arrows are named (but do not include the word "data").
- **Three-sided open rectangle (electronic or physical data storage):** Open rectangles are named and numbered (but do not include the word "file.") If more than one system shares a data store, then a **solid stripe** is placed on the left side of the rectangle to indicate this.

Collaborative Tools

SharePoint

SharePoint, a Microsoft product, is a Web-application platform that is integrated with Microsoft Office tools (e.g., Word, Excel, PowerPoint, Outlook) and can be used for content and document management, collaboration, social media, and development of websites and Intranets. SharePoint provides centralized storage of documents, which can be accessed through password-protected portals. SharePoint sites can store lists (e.g., a list of links or other similar items) and libraries (collections of documents). The SharePoint "wheel," or outcomes that SharePoint can facilitate include the following:

- Creation of sites or work environments.
- Establishment of communities, such as for sharing information or collaborating.
- Management of documents, including storing, tracking, updating, allowing collaboration, and archiving.
- Inclusion of search functions, based on keywords as well as analysis of content.
- Provision of information and insights to promote effective workflow.
- Allowance of composites and data integration.
- Templates are available for the creation of sites and subsites, and navigation is similar to that of Office products.

WebEx

WebEx, a Cisco company, provides applications that allow for internet-based videoconferencing and collaboration. WebEx products include the Cisco WebEx Meeting Center, Training Center, Support Center, and Event Center. WebEx provides a number of services, depending on the product used, including the following:

- Face-to-face internet meetings in real time.
- Notifications.
- Training for users: interactive internet training with videos and a variety of interactive tools to allow learners to participate actively in learning, including chat rooms and question and answer threads.
- Live-streaming.
- Consultation.
- Business management.
- Instant messaging.
- E-mail management.

WebEx allows participants in internet conferencing to share content, such as images and videos, in real time; thus, it allows people to collaborate at any time and from any distance, reducing the need to travel and allowing immediate consultation and videoconferencing, such as during surgery. WebEx is used for both business and education, especially for delivery of online courses or supplementary material for more traditional classes.

Wikis

Wikis are open databases that allow the user to access, edit, delete, or add material. Wikipedia, the online encyclopedia, is a well-known example of a wiki that is open to the public. Wikis can be open to anyone or can be restricted to specific groups of people; for example, a class may have a wiki to which students post information about a particular topic. Wikis may be designed for a narrow intent, such as for one class, or to manage content for a broad purpose, such as a program. Wikis may be designed with different levels of access so, for example, only certain people are allowed to delete or edit material. Wikis use simplified markup language (HTML, XML) or an online rich-text editor that allows WYSIWYG editing. Wikis support hyperlinks, and many wikis can include photos, videos, and audio files.

Blogs

Blogs are essentially online diaries or documents that are laid out in reverse chronological order (last entry viewed first) to which a blogger can add information as desired. A blog may be maintained by one person or a group of persons with shared interests. Multiauthor blogs (MABs) are becoming common. Blogs allow people to register to view the blog and to comment on entries, although they are not able to edit the blog. Blogs may contain only text, but most also have images and videos as well as links to other sites (e.g., YouTube). Blogs typically focus on one primary topic of interest, such as exercise, and some serve primarily as advertisement for companies or products. Blog-hosting services are available, although blogs can also be maintained on regular internet-hosting sites with blog software.

Social Media

Social media are internet-based programs/technology that allow users to interact with others online. Social media sites, such as Twitter, Facebook, YouTube, and LinkedIn, allow user-generated content (UGC), such as blogs, images, videos, and audio files, which are accessible by the public; however, many social media sites, such as Facebook, allow users to control access through privacy settings. PatientsLikeMe.com is a health-related website with interactivity. Internet tools used for health-related social media sites are often referred to as Health 2.0 or Medicine 2.0 and can include blogs, wikis, search functions, videocasts, and podcasts. Internet tools are increasingly used for medical education, especially in nursing curricula. Facebook is increasingly used for promotion and education by medical practitioners and other health care providers. For example, Healthcare.gov provides links to other government organizations and articles and allows users to subscribe and comment.

Project Scope and Project Plan

Project scope defines the goals of an information systems project, describing those elements to be automated and outlining both the content and the complexity. As part of the project scope, alternate solutions should be identified and feasibility considered. The project scope statement, which outlines the **project plan**, is usually done in the later stages of development as a guide for the user or consumer. The project plan should include the following:

- Objectives of the project and characteristics.
- Requirements (in terms of services and products as well as deliverables).
- Acceptance criteria.
- Limitations, boundaries, and constraints.
- Assumptions.
- Initial organization and preliminary timetable and schedule, taking into consideration the people assigned to different tasks and their skill levels.
- Identification of risks and methods to attenuate risks.
- Initial work breakdown structure, dividing the project into organized sequential steps, such as with a Gantt chart.
- Estimated costs and resources and creating a resource plan.
- Management requirements.
- Approval processes and requirements.

Concepts Related to Content Build

Computer Programming

There are five logical **steps involved in computer programming**:
1. **Problem definition**: also called function specification. The problem (or function) must be defined in detail. All contributing information necessary for solving the problem must be outlined.
2. **Program design**: Provide the functional specification: Identify what the program will do (inputs/outputs). Provide design specifications: Specific instructions for the programmer to follow.
3. **Program preparation**: The code is written in a programming language. Documents (including instructions for the user) are prepared.
4. **Program testing**: Alpha testing (also known as disk checking) is carried out by the programmers and system analyst. Beta testing (real world user testing) is carried out to check for accuracy and sufficiency.
5. **Program implementation**: Trained users test the full program (including all logical sub-routines). Programmers troubleshoot uncovered problems before the program is released.

Programming Languages

All computer software is written in a specific **programming language**. Programming languages have been divided into five separate generations based on how close they mimic human language. The first generation is binary. Binary is machine language made up of two symbols that signify off (0) and on (1). Assembler language is the second generation. Assembler language uses English letters and symbols but relates them directly to binary. For this reason, assembler language can be difficult to learn. FORTRAN, COBOL, Java, and Visual BASIC are examples of third generation programming languages. FORTRAN and COBOL are procedural languages that require the user to specify both the exact procedure to be carried out as well as the data involved. Third generation programming languages also include Java and Visual BASIC. Java is used for internet content and Visual BASIC is a visual programming language. Most people interact with computers today through fourth generation languages that allow users to choose procedures from a menu instead of having to specify them with code. In the future, it is hoped that people will be able to speak directly to computers and have them carry out the verbal commands. This will be the fifth generation of programming languages.

Structured Query Language

Structured query language (SQL) is a fourth-generation programming language (4GL) that differs from 3GLs, such as Java, in that SQL uses syntax similar to human language to access, manipulate, and retrieve data from relational database management systems, which store data in tables. Both the American National Standards Institute (ANSI) and the International Organization for Standardization have adopted SQL; however, because the language is complex, many vendors do not use the complete standard, and this limits portability between vendors without modifications. Despite many available versions, ANSI standards require that basic commands (e.g., UPDATE, DELETE, SELECT) be supported.

Language elements of SQL include the following:
- **Clauses:** from, where, group by, having, and order by
- **Expressions:** produce scales and tables
- **Predicates:** three-valued logic (null, true, false) and Boolean truth values
- **Queries:** require a SELECT statement
- **Statements:** includes the semicolon (to terminate a statement)

Programming Algorithms

There are a number of **algorithms** that are used in programming information systems. The following is a list of common algorithms and how they are applied:
- **Recursion:** Calls on itself repeatedly until a match is made. This type of algorithm is often used in functional programming.
- **Iterative:** Uses constructs that repeat themselves many times with the possible addition of other information to find a solution.
- **Logical:** Uses the controlled dedication of axioms. Algorithm = logic + control.
- **Serial:** One instruction is performed after another.
- **Parallel and Distributive:** Breaks up the algorithm into parts that can be solved on different machines and then brings the separate answers together for the results.
- **Deterministic/Non-Deterministic:** Uses precise decisions or uses a heuristically designed system of guessing.
- **Exact/Approximate:** Determines a concrete answer or determines an answer that is close enough.

The following is a **classification of programming algorithms** by the way they are designed.
- **Divide and Conquer:** Separates the problem into smaller and smaller sub-problems until each sub-problem can be solved easily.
- **Dynamic Programming:** Breaks the problem down into problems that have already been solved in order to find the answer more quickly.
- **Greedy Method:** Makes sure of approximate answers to sub-problems and can be the fastest way to find solutions.
- **Linear Programming:** Inputs are restricted based on a predetermined construct.
- **Reduction:** Changes the problem into a simpler problem.
- **Search and Enumeration:** Specifies rules in the form of a graph.

Automated Documentation

The field of nursing informatics has taken the traditional system of paper documentation and transformed it into a paperless environment using the computer system. The advantages of **automated documentation** include increased productivity due to:
- Decreases in cost, errors, and omissions.
- Improved care and communications.
- Easier access to patient information.

Paper documentation has been transformed in several different ways on a computer system including narrative charting, charting by exception, flow sheet charting, and standardized nursing languages. Narrative charting is very similar to traditional nursing documentation. It uses menu selections or text entry fields. Charting by exception allows the nurse to view normal values and change only those values for which the patient does not conform to the norm. Flow sheet charting makes use of a graphical user interface to allow the nurse to enter information from a selection of menus. Finally, standardized nursing languages use nationally and internationally defined codes to enter information free from ambiguity.

Layout

Developing screens for consistency and ease of use requires an understanding of the basic **layout** and text guidelines. Headings should be placed uppermost and in the same place on subsequent screens. The eye should move in a continuous line (usually top to bottom), so images and text should not be scattered about a page but arranged in an orderly vertical display. Bright colors are distracting, and red and green should be avoided because some people may be color blind to those colors. Complex images and illustrations are difficult to view on the screen, so simple designs are preferable. Menu and status bars should be in the same place on each screen (usually top or bottom) and should contain only essential items. Icons should be easily recognizable and consistent. Unnecessary lines on the screen, such as borders, should be avoided.

Text

Text is more tiring for the eyes on the screen than on the printed page because of the illumination of the screen, and some fonts may blur in browsers, so fonts especially designed for the internet, such as Verdana and Lucida Sans/Grande, should be used for text that will be accessed by a browser. Using a variety of fonts and multiple sizes on one screen can be very distracting. Long paragraphs should be avoided, and information should be presented in small paragraphs with adequate white space to rest the eyes. Font size should be 12–14 for standard text with larger sizes for headings. Text against a colored background, especially a deep color, is difficult to read. When highlighting text, underlining is more evident than italicizing and bolding because screens have different lighting and resolution. Colored fonts may be used sparingly to highlight different types of information. For example, a question or heading may be in a blue font and an explanation in a black font.

Designing Systems to Support Workflow

Human-Centered Design

The following steps are required for **human-centered design**:
1. Define and understand the organization's requirements and the requirements of the individual users.
2. Define and understand the logistics of how and where the system will be used.
3. Perform a functionality analysis. Specific system tasks should be broken down by priority, duration, frequency, and probability of completion.
4. Define the key system functions. The system functions should be logical and intuitive to the end users.
5. Perform an analysis of the most common potential errors that could occur during tasks. Minimize the likelihood of committing errors by optimizing processes.
6. Design interfaces and workstations so that they will work best with the users.
7. Perform system testing with actual users. Depending on the results of these tests, the system should be adjusted to create the best system for the users.

Ergonomics

Ergonomics is the study of the work environment and its effect on humans. There are three types of ergonomics:
- **Physical:** Physical ergonomics deals with the interaction between a person's body and a machine.
- **Cognitive:** Cognitive ergonomics (also known as engineering psychology) deals with the interaction between the human mind and work.
- **Organized:** Organized ergonomics (also known as macro ergonomics) deals with the culture of work including issues of safety and ethics.

When implementing a new information system in a medical facility, it is important to consider all three types of ergonomics. First, the interactive devices (e.g., computer screens and keyboards) must be physically easy to work with and have a low risk of physical injury. Second, the staff must be psychologically willing to value the new computer system and use it effectively. Finally, the ethical use of the system must be defined and written standards put in place to assure consistency.

Findings of Current Ergonomics Research

The user of the ergonomic device has to be evaluated along with the equipment and setting. All humans are different and have different ergonomic needs. The best ergonomic solution for one individual may not necessarily work for another. It should also be noted that the workstation may not appear to be configured in the best way to the supervisor (or casual observer), but may indeed be the best for the user.

There is no such thing as a true ergonomic chair. Chairs are manufactured with many adjustable features. Some of these are effective and some are not. Chairs should be chosen that would accommodate the widest variety of users (body types) that will be sitting on them. Additionally, chair parts and padding wear out very quickly. What may have once begun as a very suitable ergonomic chair could deteriorate into a poor choice in a relatively short amount of time. Used chairs should be refurbished or disposed.

Repetitive Stress Injury and Carpal Tunnel Syndrome

Repetitive stress injury: Any injury resulting from performing a similar motion repeatedly. In the late 1990's, there was a large increase in repetitive stress (motion) injuries reported by healthcare workers due to the increased use of computers and other electronic devices.

Carpal tunnel syndrome: This is the most well-known repetitive stress injury. It involves the compression of the median nerve located in the wrist. It is usually seen in individuals who spend many hours in front of a computer screen typing. Ergonomic keyboards and wrist rests have not been shown to significantly decrease the chance of developing carpal tunnel syndrome. Many sufferers do report relief when using wrist splints at night to rest their affected hand(s). One of the best ways to keep from developing carpal tunnel syndrome is to take frequent breaks from the keyboard or mouse and perform simple exercises designed to alleviate pressure on the median nerve. Once carpal tunnel syndrome has been diagnosed, it can be treated with steroid injections, anti-inflammatory medications, or (less commonly) surgery.

Ergonomically Designed Computer Workstations

The following are some important **ergonomic factors** in regards to the design of computer workstations:
- Deciding how it will be used: How will the user interface with the information system?
- Finding out how long the user will be in place: How many hours will the user be stationed at the interface? Is the time continuous?
- Configured based on the equipment to be used: Does the user have to turn or reach for various components of the information system during their routine operations?
- Located in areas of low noise: Is the noise environment conducive to the tasks the user needs to perform?
- Located in areas of good ventilation: Are environmental conditions appropriate for the users and equipment?
- Use stable workstation furniture: Is the workstation furniture suitable for the equipment that it supports?
- Educate users on proper usage: Do the users follow the proper ergonomic procedures for performing their job?
- Choose chairs with proper back support: Is the user's chair appropriate for the user in terms of adjustability and back support?

Enhancing the Ergonomics of a User Workstation

Due to the danger of repetitive motion stress injuries and other hazards of working with computers, designers have developed a number of ergonomic enhancement products to be used in the computer work environment. They are:
- **Glare filter:** This helps reduce eyestrain from light reflecting from a user's monitor.
- **Negative keyboard angles:** This allows the keyboard to be situated below the elbows and allows the wrists to be held at a straighter, more natural angle.
- **Document holder:** This holds documents at eye level so that the user may type and enter information without moving their neck up and down.

- **Lumbar support:** This helps support the back more comfortably, and helps position the back with a proper curvature to alleviate stress.
- **Footrest:** This helps to improve posture, increase blood flow to the feet, and prevent lower back pain.

Ergonomically Designed Keyboards

There are three major types of **ergonomically designed keyboards**:
- **Split keyboard:** This type of keyboard was designed to minimize the occurrence of the hand and wrist position that places pressure on the major nerves in the wrist. There are two types of split keyboard designs; one directs each keyboard half out toward the elbows while the other completely separates the keyboard so that the halves can be located in-line with the elbows.
- **Tented keyboards** are similarly split into two halves; however, they also allow the typist to angle their palms toward one another reducing the joint posture known as pronation.
- **Negative-slope keyboards** were developed to reduce wrist extension by allowing the user to tilt the keyboard to a flat or backward slope opposite of the more traditional positive slope keyboard.

Ergonomic research results for these keyboards are mixed, with individuals who already have ulnar nerve damage receiving the most benefit.

Supportive, Scooped Key, Minimum-Motion, and Straight Column Keyboards

There are a number of alternative keyboards on the market:
- **Supportive keyboards.** These keyboards have a built in wrist rest. While the wrist rest may help the individual user sit with a more comfortable posture, it may also allow fluid to build up in the carpal tunnel causing wrist pain.
- **Scooped key arrangement keyboards.** These keyboards are designed in bowl-like shapes. This type of design has the keys set closer together which allows for an extra row of keys. The intent is to reduce reach fatigue.
- **Minimum-motion keyboards.** These keyboards were developed to change the way the individual keys are operated. Rather than pushing the keys down flat (as is the case with traditional keyboards), the user only has to lightly touch them. This is meant to reduce muscle tension and finger pain.
- **Straight column keyboards.** This keyboard places keys running straight up and down instead of in diagonally offset rows (as is the case for traditional keyboards). This arrangement helps to lessen stress on the left hand with little effect on the right hand.

Ergonomic Chairs

The following are main features of a good **ergonomic chair**:
- The ability to adjust the height of the seat. Preferably, this should include a pneumatic adjuster that allows a customized setting rather than a ratcheting mechanism. The user should be able to adjust the chair so that their thighs are parallel to the floor (with both feet flat on the floor).
- The ability to adjust seat pad front-to-back. This will allow individuals of different heights to support their legs and feel comfortable.

- The chair should have padded armrests that are adjustable for both height and width. This will prevent arm strain by providing passive support of the elbows. The forearms and hands will then be in the correct neutral position for typing.
- The chair should be able to recline to transfer some upper body weight to the backrest.
- The chair should have an adjustable back support to prevent lumbar compression.

Alleviating the Detrimental Effects of Prolonged Mouse Use and Prolonged Sitting

Prolonged mouse usage can lead to pain and nerve damage in the wrist, hand, and fingers. Solutions known to help include:
- Adhere to a break schedule that allows you to stretch and rest your hands and arms.
- Alternate the hand that uses the mouse (e.g., if you are left handed, switch the mouse to your right hand).
- Perform a wider variety of work that involves more than sitting behind a desk.
- Use an ergonomically designed alternative to a mouse (such as a track ball).
- Use keystroke substitutes to avoid repetitive motion.

Prolonged sitting can place strain on the back that may lead to pain and nerve damage. The following is a list of solutions that are known to help:
- Adhere to a schedule that allows you to stand up, walk, and stretch.
- Use an adjustable chair to maintain a good posture.
- Place equipment (such as a phone or printer) so that it forces you to get out of your chair.
- Consider a workstation that allows you the flexibility to sit or stand and perform your work.

Americans with Disabilities Act

The 1992 **Americans with Disabilities Act (ADA)** is civil rights legislation that provides the disabled, including those with mental impairment, access to employment and the community. The ADA prevents discrimination against employees or potential employees for organizations with fifteen or more employees because of disabilities. The Equal Employment Opportunity Commission enforces these provisions. Employers are only allowed to ask applicants if they need accommodations, not if they have disabilities, and individual accommodations must be made. Accommodations can include the following:
- Alterations in work station
- Speech recognition software
- Screen magnifying software
- Optical character recognition systems
- Video captioning
- Braille readers and screen readers
- Adapted keyboards and on-screen keyboard
- Teletypewriter or text display device
- Amplification systems

People who are disabled are entitled to assistive technology that will allow them to function but are not entitled to jobs that they are unable to do even with assistive devices or accommodations. Most computer operating systems now incorporate assistive technology (e.g., screen readers).

Systems Implementation

System Implementation Strategies

System implementation begins early by preparing staff and users for changes. An implementation committee should be formed before purchase of a system to assess needs and ensure that changes meet the mission of the organization. Nurses should have an active role in the implementation committee, which must develop a project plan and timetable. Project planning software is available to develop a work breakdown structure, which is a plan with a timeline and breakdown of specific tasks. Committee members must be educated about the system so they can serve as resources during the extensive training that needs to occur before implementation. Factors to consider during selection of an information system include the currency of the technology, the ability to upgrade, and issues related to obsolescence, vendor history, vendor compliance with regulations, ability to integrate with existing or other systems, flexibility, support of electronic health records, and the computer data source. Hardware analysis includes network infrastructure, types of workstations/devices, hardware locations, and printing capabilities and locations.

Phased Implementation

Phased implementation of a new system may involve phasing by module, unit, or geography. In phased implementation, the system may go live in one or more units initially with units added on an extended phased schedule until all units have switched to the new system. This has the advantage of allowing for evaluation and revision on a small scale. Additionally, those initially using the new system may subsequently serve as trainers and resources for those who receive the system at a later time. In some cases of phased implementation, some aspects of a new system may be used throughout the organization with other aspects added in phased steps. For example, all units may be able to retrieve data but only some to enter data. Careful consideration should be given to which units should receive the new system first. It is usually best to begin with people with computer skills or those who support the new system. Disadvantages include disruption of operations, difficulty in accessing complete data, and staff confusion.

Big-Bang Implementation

Big-bang implementation occurs when a complete system goes live across an organization on a designated date and time. For example, if the prior system involved paper documentation, this stops, and all entries are done on the new computerized system. The big-bang approach is best in small organizations where people have been well trained in the new system, have competent computer skills, or have mentors readily available. A phased approach may be better for a large organization because inevitable problems arise during transition. Lists of those who are trained and can assist others should be published, and training should be a staffing consideration so that all units have mentors available. All data must be converted from the old system into the new system before implementation, and the validity of the data must be verified because errors can occur during conversion. Advantages are rapid change, less updating of documentation, and focused training. Disadvantages include confusion, lost data, learning curve, and startup problems. Fallback plans should be in place in the event of system failure.

Pilot Implementation

Pilot implementation is often used in large organizations or those with multiple locations to "try out" the new system before it is implemented further. This is similar to phased implementation except that it is usually limited to one or few units, and extensive evaluation is usually completed during the pilot program. This evaluation includes interviews with users to determine what faults exist and assessment of end-user acceptance so that any alterations or modifications can be completed before further implementation. With pilot implementation, initial training may be restricted to those in the pilot program. The early adopters may be used as trainers and mentors in later implementation. Pilot programs are often easiest to assess in stand-alone units that do not require a lot of data transmission to and from other units.

Parallel Implementation

In **parallel implementation**, both the existing (legacy) system and new system are used concurrently; for example, when moving from paper charting to computerized record keeping, both systems are used. A timetable is usually established for phasing out the legacy system. Parallel implementation allows end-users to learn the new system while still using the old system to record data. This method is usually faster than phased implementation but slower than big bang and tends to be the most costly both in terms of finances and time, as users must enter data in two systems, increasing the risks of errors. However, this format does allow for evaluation of the accuracy of use of the new system, as comparison data are available in the legacy system. Parallel implementation is also less risky in terms of system failure than big bang implementation because a backup system is essentially in place.

Formation of an Implementation Team

The following steps are needed to form an **effective implementation** team:
Step 1: Select a leader who will own the implementation process.
Step 2: Form the team with representation from the various users of the system (e.g., IT staff, executives, and nurses)
Step 3: To assure success, look for the following team member characteristics:
- Good communication skills
- Can multi-task effectively
- Good cooperation in the team environment
Step 4: Keep the team focused on the final goal of implementing an effective system.

Role of the Informatics Nurse (Business Integrator) in the Implementation of Information Systems

When a new information system is going to be **implemented, the informatics nurse** (or business integrator) is in a particularly important position to support the process. For this role, the following items should be included in the implementation plan:
- A statement of support from the upper management of the company.
- An assessment on how the new system will impact the various jobs that will be within the scope of the implementation.
- A complete overview of the implementation plan and the methods being used.
- An assessment on how the new system will affect the company culture (particularly nursing).
- A budget that includes where the money will come from and how this will affect finances.

Individuals Who Should Be Included on the Steering Committee of an Information System Implementation

It is important when implementing a new information system into the clinical environment to have **representatives** from all areas of the organization that will be affected by the new system, including those listed below:

- **Hospital Administration**: In order to assure that business processes are maintained.
- **Finance**: To assure that billing and patient records are maintained, in addition to establishing a budget.
- **Nurse administrator**: To facilitate that nursing procedures are compatible with the new system.
- **Director of the Information Systems department**: To oversee that the system is installed properly.
- **Medical records**: To assure that record keeping is accurate and follows all regulatory requirements (e.g., HIPAA)

Assignment of Resources

Assigning resources involves understanding the types of resources available—educational, personnel, financial, and equipment—as each must be allocated, using different priorities; therefore, establishing a list of priorities for each category of resources is essential. Prioritizing may be done by the informatics nurse specialist alone or with guidance from an advisory committee. For example, educational resources, such as computerized modules, videos, and texts, may first be assigned to those in a particular unit where training is essential. Personnel should be assigned, according to need, in terms of actual number of staff, work time, and duration of time. Financial allocation includes ongoing costs of maintaining a system, costs of updates and enhancements, and contingency costs (e.g., when problems arise or equipment malfunctions). Equipment resources, such as handheld devices and biometric monitoring devices, are allocated according to need, which is often determined by an advisory committee.

System Enhancements

The availability of **system enhancements**, such as software upgrades, new software, and new hardware, is almost constant, but constant changes to a system can result in changes in functionality and a need for increased resources and training. A committee that reviews requests for enhancements can help to determine which are needed by the organization and which are unnecessary. Enhancements should be evaluated in terms of impact on efficiency and cost-effectiveness. Introducing enhancements to a system that change functionality requires advance notice to staff and, sometimes, additional training, so holding the introduction of enhancements to a schedule, such as every 6 weeks, may be less disruptive than routinely updating software and equipment as updates become available. Testing the enhancement should be completed, when possible, before wide dissemination.

System Implementation Process

The following steps are involved in administering **the system implementation process**:

- **Step 1:** Develop a schedule (with strategic milestones) that will be used to install the new system. This is sometimes referred to as the work breakdown structure (WBS) of the project.

- **Step 2:** Assign tasks. These tasks should be specific, assigned to capable persons, and tracked (for completion).
- **Step 3:** Establish a communications plan that covers the methods and timing of all communication within and outside of the implementation team.
- **Step 4:** Test the system (in a controlled test environment) before going live. This gives the users and a support staff opportunity to stress the system and assure that it is operating properly.

Upgrading or Implementing Information Systems

The following steps are necessary whenever an organization is **upgrading** or implementing an information system:
- Planning and administration of the project: Establish the planning and project teams, and set the key milestones for the project.
- Delivery of hardware and software: Select the vendor and purchase the hardware and software.
- Program installation: Provide time for installation and perform a qualification (system testing, interfaces to databases, etc.) of the newly installed components.
- Policies and procedures: Develop and approve the relevant policies and procedures.
- Training: Provide training for all relevant personnel.
- Maintenance and support: Set up a maintenance and user support procedure.

Making Recommendations for Programming Changes

Programming changes are common with information systems because of updates, upgrades, and the addition of new features. Technology is constantly changing along with user needs and regulatory requirements, so programming must accommodate these changes. Typically, software upgrades are released on an 18-month schedule, and often one upgrade can be skipped without a significant impact on productivity; however, by the third year, obsolescence is an issue, and upgrading and making necessary programming changes are usually necessary, so management must carefully assess the value of upgrades, needs of the organization, and associated time and costs in implementation when making recommendations. Changes in regulatory requirements may occur every year or 2, so monitoring requirements and making necessary programming changes are essential.

Resistance to Organizational Change

Performance improvement processes cannot occur without organizational change, and **resistance to change** is common for many people, so coordinating collaborative processes requires anticipating resistance and taking steps to achieve cooperation. Resistance often relates to concerns about job loss, increased responsibilities, and general denial or lack of understanding and frustration. Leaders can prepare others involved in the process of change by taking these steps:
- Be honest, informative, and tactful, giving people thorough information about anticipated changes and how the changes will affect them, including positives.
- Be patient in allowing people the time they need to contemplate changes and express anger or disagreement.
- Be empathetic in listening carefully to the concerns of others.
- Encourage participation, allowing staff to propose methods of implementing change, so they feel some sense of ownership.

- Establish a climate in which all staff members are encouraged to identify the need for change on an ongoing basis.
- Present further ideas for change to management.

Hardware Infrastructure Analysis

The following **hardware infrastructure requirements** should be evaluated and satisfied before the new system is installed:
- Network infrastructure: cable/wireless local area network (LAN) installation, available access points, and overall compatibility with the new system.
- The type(s) of user workstation interfaces (desktop computer, laptop computer, terminals, etc.).
- The location of the workstations (portable or permanent).
- The physical location of the hardware (servers).
- The connectivity and location of printers and/or other output devices.

Back Loading Existing Data into a New Information System

The following steps are involved in the **back loading of data** into a new information system:
- Decide what information needs to be migrated to the new system.
- Establish who is responsible for entering the existing data into the new system.
- Set a schedule for the timing of the data transfer.
- Establish the time frame for migration of historical data.
- Implement controls to assure that all back loaded information is accurate.
- Verify that the system is working properly.

Anticipated Problems That May Occur During Implementation of a New System

The following **problems** may occur when introducing a new information system into a healthcare facility:
- Failing to allocate adequate time for system implementation.
- Scope creep: allowing the project to exceed the original scope (e.g., adding extra features or functions without paying attention to timeline or budget). This tends to occur slowly during the conduct of the project and ultimately results in exceeding the budget and/or timeline.
- Allowing programmers to customize a system beyond what is necessary.
- Not allowing enough funds for maintenance.
- Failing to provide dedicated staff to work on the project.
- Encountering organizational resistance to change that causes roadblocks or delays.
- Not allowing enough time to adequately test the system.
- Not allowing enough time to train relevant staff.

Planning the "Go-Live" Process

Set the date when the system is anticipated to **go-live** and whether the system will be scaled up in a staggered (according to certain client types), modular (according to facility or department) or an all at once manner.

Create an overall implementation strategy that includes:
- Transfer of data from the old system to the new system.
- Establish a user and system support system.
- Develop the various short- and long-term evaluation procedures to monitor the new system.
- Develop a change control procedure to assure that all changes to the new system are documented and carried out properly.

The **final stages** of a **go-live implementation** are:
- Establish a user support structure and its format (phone, internet-based, etc.).
- Develop a procedure for change control regarding changes to the system and future upgrades/maintenance.
- The go-live period is a very labor-intensive period for project personnel. A work schedule (including any necessary overtime) should be created in anticipation of this expected workload.
- An implementation feedback loop for users should be created. This may consist of paper questionnaires, a dedicated phone number/e-mail address, or a website.
- A permanent committee should be established to review requests and implement changes.

Data Conversion/Migration

Data conversion/migration occurs when data are translated from one format to another. During implementation of a new system, data migration must occur for the new system to use legacy data but may also occur during system hardware/software upgrades. Migration usually requires software (commercial or in-house) as well as manual effort. The primary stages to migration of data include:
- **Planning stage:** This includes inventorying the system, reviewing the types and amounts of data to be migrated and the source and destination formats, determining the most cost-effective method, making a specific plan for conversion, performing mapping, and creating conversion scripts and specification documents.
- **Performance stage:** This includes generating baseline backup of all data, extracting data from the source, normalizing data, performing trial and test conversions, and completing data migration.
- **Validation stage:** This includes checking to ensure data were converted accurately and completely with all data elements formatted correctly, eliminating duplicate data, and resolving problems.

Interoperability

Interoperability is the ability for two systems to exchange and use data while maintaining the same meaning, and this is an important element in the conversion of data. Types of interoperability include the following:
- **Technical interoperability** refers to the ability of two systems or equipment from different manufacturers to exchange data. This usually refers to hardware/software or equipment that allows machine-to-machine communication.
- **Syntactical interoperability** refers to the transfer of data formats without necessarily ensuring that meaning is intact.

- **Semantic interoperability** refers to the transfer of meaning so that people recognize that the content transferred is the same.
- **Process interoperability** refers to processes and specifications that facilitate exchange of data from one organization to another.

Noninteroperability may result from lack of adequate system review, changes in standards that interfere with the application to another system, and varying levels of technical quality from one system to another.

Archiving Legacy Data

Systems often contain large amounts of obsolete legacy data; however, keeping an old system running to allow access to the data is expensive, but moving all data to the new system may result in huge amounts of data posing problems in translation. A cost-effective solution is to **archive legacy data** to archive appliances, which offload data from the main storage system in an accessible format (online or offline). When determining which data are to remain active and which are to be decommissioned, the processes include:
- Evaluating and auditing the data to eliminate redundancies.
- Determining what data are important for business/legal reasons.
- Evaluating data to determine what should be active and inactive.
- Evaluating legal requirements in relationship to data.
- Reviewing the organizational policies regarding data retention.
- Developing a plan for archiving and decommissioning data.
- Validating the integrity of the data.

Command Center

During the conversion and go-live process, a **command center**, comprised of a director and support staff, can coordinate and monitor all operations (e.g., applications, user support, vendor support, communication, documentation, technical operations). The command center should be established as part of the preliminary planning. Three primary functions of the command center include:
- **Providing communication** to all parties and evaluating intelligence regarding problems.
- **Exercising control** over the process of conversion, allocating resources appropriately, and demonstrating leadership in advocating for change.
- **Coordinating all activities** and **maintaining documentation**.

Members of the command center should be in the same area or adjacent areas to allow for fast and effective communication. Vendor representatives may be at the center and at off-site locations and are often critical during the go-live procedures.

Data Dictionary and Master Patient Index

In order to integrate computer systems, two major items of importance are the data dictionary and a master patient index. These two items need to be recognized by the various systems that make up the integrated system. In computing, recognition means that the data have to be similar in structure and characters.

- **Data dictionary:** A data dictionary lists commonly used terms, their definition, and their synonyms. It should also list the term that should be used by all departments as the de facto standard in order to facilitate integration.
- **Master patient index:** The master patient index (MPI) lists all patients and their demographic information. It is important that each individual be listed with several different pieces of data including: first and last name, social security number, and date of birth. The MPI should be set up so that new fields of information can be added easily and that it can be scaled up (without slowing down system performance) as the business grows.

Computer System Integration

Within a company, the need for an **integrated computer system** is necessary. Companies may choose to switch from many separate systems to one integrated system, or may invest in a computer interface program that will decode information between separate systems. The advantage of having an integrated system is that information is automatically transferred between the various independent systems that make up the parts of the integrated system. This results in a more robust, less error prone, combined system. There are two major types of interfaces:

- **Point-to-point:** The point-to-point interface connects two separate systems directly to each other.
- **Software reliance systems:** For systems that need to interface with more than two entities, it is best to use an interface engine software. This results in a more flexible network. Interface engine software can process information in real-time or in batches. Real-time processing means that information is transferred from one system to another immediately. Batch processing occurs at the end of the day when all information is transferred at one time.

Testing

System Testing

Before going live with a hospital information system, the system should be thoroughly tested to assure that it is operating properly. This is accomplished by performing a **system test plan.** The system test plan consists of the following four steps:

- **Step 1:** Develop the overall test plan. This includes the installation, operation, and validation of the new system.
- **Step 2:** Create the test scripts. These are the scripts that actual users of the system will use to "stress" the system to determine if it is working according to specifications. They should reflect real use as closely as possible.
- **Step 3:** Carry out the testing and troubleshoot and system's failings as soon as possible.

Feasibility Study

A **feasibility study** will help to define the problem(s) that the new information system is expected to address. It will also answer questions regarding cost, goals, and specific outcomes. Some specific questions may include:

- How will the outcome (e.g., meeting the pre-defined business requirements) be measured?
- What research has been done to back up the proposal?
- What are the risks in terms of people, money, and time?
- How long will the implementation take and what will be involved?
- Will the project require dedicated staff members, contractors, or a combination of both?

Components

Components are software applications, such as those commercially available or prepared by third parties, which need to be integrated into the other software of the information system. Testing is completed to determine if the software meets specifications and functions properly and whether it meets interaction requirements of the system. Tests verify if specific areas of code work correctly. Factors to consider include the ease with which the software's functions can be observed, behavior traceability, the difficulty or ease of functions and operations, and the method the component uses to provide or present information. Components may be tested by the developer and by the user, but the user may lack the source codes necessary for effective testing. In some cases, if software is functioning well, further testing may not be indicated. In general, those components that should be tested include reusable and domain components. Commercial components are often reusable and should be tested and evaluated for liability issues. When possible, reusable testing strategies should be developed.

Features

Features are parts of a component with predictable properties. Systems have become increasingly complex because of the expansion in features. Feature creep is the term used to describe the addition of more and more features to a program. Features may relate to data, hardware, software, end-users, and telecommunications and facilitate the four primary functions of an information system: allowing input, providing storage, processing data, and providing output.

Features may include the following:

- Management of database (e.g., storage, retrieval, import, export).
- Ability to generate reports.
- Ability to integrate with other components of a system and scalability.
- E-mail and other customizable alerts.
- Time keeping/login and logout times.
- Communication among different levels and multisite capabilities.
- Real-time processing.
- Ability to establish uniform procedures.
- Ability to provide feedback.

Interface

Interface is a computer program that allows two or more programs to exchange information. If the connection is direct, the interface is point-to-point and allows transfer of data only between two programs. Interface engine software allows information to transfer from one system to a number of different systems. In this case, translation tables move data from the clinical data repository (collective database) to each system. Because terms may vary from one system to another, mapping is required to associate terms in one system with comparable terms in other systems. The serial peripheral interface bus (SPI) is a *de facto* industry standard, although different vendors have different configurations. SPI allows master/slave communication from the master device to single or multiple slave devices. SPI is full duplex and facilitates communication in both directions simultaneously. Half duplex interfaces facilitate communication in both directions but only in one direction at a time. SPI is used to communicate with a variety of peripheral devices, such as sensors, clocks, liquid-crystal displays, universal serial bus ports, and communications (e.g., Ethernet, handheld devices).

User Interface

A **user interface** (human–computer/machine interface) allows interaction between the user and the machine (e.g., computer, other electronic devices), permitting the user to make input and to see output as a result. The design of this interface must consider the needs of the user and ease of use. Types of current and new interfaces include the following:

- **Touch screens and touch user:** Often used in simulations, the device has a combined use of input and output.
- **Graphical user:** This allows an interface between devices, such as the keyboard and computer. It includes object-oriented user interfaces as well as application-oriented interfaces.
- **Gesture:** This allows input from gestures and mouse/stylus movements.
- **Zooming:** This allows changes in scale of output.
- **Voice user:** Input is by keystrokes or voice commands, and output is by voice commands.
- **Natural language:** This allows input by keystrokes in natural language (e.g., questions), and output is the response.
- **Zero-input:** Input derives from sensors.

Links

Links (i.e., highlighted words, icons, images) allow access of information at one point from a different point. For example, a link may allow the user to jump from one part of a document to another or one document to another. In some cases, links may be external, such as links to websites. When the user clicks on a link, a transmission control protocol/internet protocol connection is established between the user and server, resulting in a hypertext transfer protocol request of information. All links must be tested individually to ensure they function properly. Links may open in different ways, such as in a popup window or by replacing the content of the original window. Links may be generated automatically, such as with alerts, or accessed manually.

Devices

Devices include input devices, such as keyboards, mouse, microphone, stylus, webcams, and output devices, such as terminals, printers, projectors, and screens. The informatics nurse specialist must understand the system architecture and how all of the devices are interconnected as well as how the operating system interfaces with the devices. Other necessary information includes the configuration of the individual devices and software access as well as the manner in which to add individual devices to an existing system. Different operating systems use different naming protocols for similar devices and display information about devices in different manners. Devices can be in four different states when connected to a system:

- **Undefined:** The system does not recognize the device.
- **Defined:** Information about a specific device is present in the database but not available to the system.
- **Available:** Information about a device is present in the database and configured to the operating system.
- **Not available/stopped:** Information about the device is present in its driver, but the device is not available.

Reports

Information systems provide a number of different types of **reports**, and these should be assessed for accuracy. Some reports are generated automatically, and others require manual input to define the type of report and information needed. Types of reports that may be available include:

- **Configuration:** These reports contain data about the system itself, including hardware and software, as well as workstations and servers. Configuration reports may be generated by systems or data sets.
- **Informational:** Often informational reports include built-in templates and provide fact-finding to glean information from databases.
- **Change:** Usually change reports are automated, showing changes that occur in the system over a period of time.
- **Baseline:** Usually baseline reports are automated to show how the system or elements of the system compare to a baseline.
- **Summary/management:** These reports show summaries of actions, processes, and data.
- **Periodic:** Periodic reports are issued at predetermined periods, such as monthly claims reports.
- **Error/exception:** Error or exception reports are issued when faults occur or data are outside of normal parameters.

Screens

Screens, such as those on computer monitors, smartphones, or tablets, display both text and graphic images. Early computer screens used cathode ray technology (CRT), but this has been almost completely replaced by liquid crystal display (LCD) technology, used for flat panel displays. LCDs have a lower power demand than CRTs or plasma displays (used primarily for large screen televisions); additionally, they are more lightweight and smaller. LCDs have two sheets of polarizing material with a liquid crystal solution between the sheets. For touch screen capabilities or use of a stylus, an electromagnetic field is added. Considerations include:

- **Refresh rate:** This is the speed at which the screen reprints from top to bottom. Slow refresh rates on CRTs can cause flickering, but this does not occur with LCDs, which have a frame rate (the rate at which consecutive images or frames appear) expressed in frames per second, usually about 60.
- **Resolution:** This is the number of horizontal pixels by vertical, such as 1440 x 900. The higher the resolution, the clearer (but smaller) the image.

Systems Environment

The **systems environment** is assessed through analysis of the internal environment (e.g., staff, physicians, board) and external environment (e.g., vendors, patients, agencies). A needs assessment may be required to determine the type of data required. Data may be derived from the following:

- Published materials (e.g., journal articles, reports)
- Vendor materials (e.g., pamphlets, specifications)
- Organizational input
- Regulatory requirements
- Accreditation requirements
- Marketing trends
- Interviews and questionnaires
- Technological trends

Data are analyzed to identify trends, needs, and expectations. Once potential actions or solutions to problems are identified, they must be further analyzed and comparisons made, considering the needs of end-users. After implementation of a system, ongoing testing, analysis, and feedback are necessary to ensure that needs are met and that the system functions effectively.

Automated Testing

Automated testing involves using software tools specifically designed to test features of an information system, such as the graphical user interface (GUI). Automated testing does not require manual intervention. The software may include tools to provide comparison data regarding expected and actual outcomes and well as other reports. Automated testing often mimics the actions of users, but automated testing must include adequate testing scripts to be used effectively. Applications may include program monitors, debugging tools, GUI testing tools, profiling tools (to generate reports), and benchmarks. Metrics (standards of measurement) must be developed to address performance issues, and the goals and expected outcomes of automated testing should be clearly defined. Automated testing is especially valuable in the types of testing that may not be practical to do manually, such as stress testing in which a system is tested with large numbers of simulated users.

Unit/Component (Suitability Testing Methods)

Unit or component suitability testing methods include:
- Black box – This is a form of functional testing that determines if an input results in the correct output, using test cases focused on the system's operational profile. This type of testing does not require knowledge of code or inner product design. Testing may not include activation of all codes, so it may not detect all faults.
- Fault injection – This introduces faults into the system to show what happens to the system when the component fails to function properly.
- Operational system – This tests the ability of the system to function after introduction of a component. However, this may require a huge amount of testing to determine how the system will deal with component failures or problems.
- Defense building – Wrappers are used to limit the component software in some way; that is, the wrapper may check or limit input into the component or check or limit output to the system. Wrappers are often employed when commercial software is purchased that only partially meets requirements.

System Integration Testing

System integration testing (SIT), part of software/hardware testing, determines if hardware or software applications can work together. Integration testing is done after unit testing and before system and acceptance testing and involves testing how all the units function together. This is a type of black box testing that should not require knowledge of code or inner product design. The purpose of the testing is to identify problems or faults within the component parts (assemblages) or within the entire information system that affects performance. SIT may include load, volume, and usability testing. SIT involves development of an integration test plan that outlines what will be tested and how the tests will be conducted as well as pass/fail criteria. Test cases may be developed to identify transitions and present end-user scenarios. Test data should be developed to use in the test cases. Approaches to integration testing include big bang (includes all components), top down (higher level components before lower level), and bottom up (lower level components before higher level).

Functional Testing

Functional testing verifies that a code is functioning properly and determines if users are able to carry out certain functions or whether features in the software work as expected. Functional testing may include manipulating data, conducting searches, using user commands, and accessing user screens. Integration testing is also conducted as part of functional testing. Functional testing should be completed on units during development and on the system as a whole after integration. Functional testing should also be conducted from the perspective of the end-user, so functional tests should always be designed to correspond to end-user requirements. Functional testing may include both manual and automated testing components. Functional tests should be able to identify system level faults and problems.

Load, or Volume Testing

Load, or **volume testing**, is a type of nonfunctional reliability testing that evaluates the system's ability to function under different loads, such as during normal use times and peak times with multiple users to determine maximum capacity and problems that might be encountered. This test involves evaluating the effect of volume on the system to determine limits. Testing tries to

Copyright © Mometrix Media. You have been licensed one copy of this document for personal use only. Any other reproduction or redistribution is strictly prohibited. All rights reserved.

determine at which exact point problems arise. This can include static and dynamic testing of the system at the safe working load (SWL) and above the SWL. Volume testing may include testing the ability of an application to handle a certain volume of data, such as in a database. Volume testing should always be concluded before a system becomes live to prevent crashes and loss of data if limits are exceeded.

Validating Data Integration Across Disparate Systems

Validating data integration across disparate systems is essential because incorrect data can lead to serious problems with the system and provide false information. Validating every item of data is virtually impossible, but doing spot checks of representative data may miss faults. Validation should include assessing the size of data, including the number of files or records, before and after data transfer to a disparate system to ensure it is the same and that the data source is completely transferred correctly. Data should be complete, accurate, and formatted correctly, and duplicate elements should be eliminated. Important elements of validation include:
- Validating across all levels of data, determining frequency, duration, and areas of applications.
- Validating at high granularity (degree of breakdown into smaller units/parts) rather than low.
- Validating data that are especially critical.
- Automating validation.
- Thoroughly understanding the source of data as well as its input and storage.
- Customizing validation approaches, according to the needs of the organization.

Analysis of Systems Performance Effectiveness and Accessibility

Systems testing for **performance effectiveness** is completed after integration testing and involves testing the system as a whole to determine if it meets requirements, functions as needed, and meets expected outcomes. Numerous tests are involved in systems testing.

Accessibility—Testing is completed to ensure that the system is in compliance with the ADA requirements. This includes testing speech recognition software, screen magnifying software, video captioning, braille readers, amplification systems, alternative keyboards, and screen readers to determine if they function properly through various actions. Technical compliance with requirements of the Federal Electronic and Information Technology Accessibility and Compliance Act (1997) must also be tested where applicable. Testing should also be done to ensure that internet access is in compliance with standards set by the Web Accessibility Initiative (WAI), which provides guidelines to allow those with disabilities to access the internet and create content.

Ad hoc—This type of exploratory testing is usually done once, and the user attempts to identify problems in an unstructured way by trying various means to elicit errors. This is essentially a form of error guessing in which the user bases testing on previous experience with software.

Compatibility—This may include certification testing to determine if the application functions properly in a target operating system or database. Compatibility testing, focusing on user experience, can encompass a wide range of tests, such as testing the system in different web browsers, evaluating the bandwidth handling capacity, determining if peripherals (e.g., printers) function properly, evaluating the function of tools (e.g., messaging), and testing access to databases.

Exception handling—This type of error testing is done to determine if there are errors resulting from incorrect programming, coding, or resource failures, how the system responds, and whether errors result in negative effects, such as corrupted data. Exception handling may involve hardware and software.

Exploratory—This type of testing uses the results of previous testing to determine the types of additional testing indicated, based on user experience, and does not follow a specified pattern of testing. This may be done after conclusion of other tests to verify that no significant defects remain.

Graphical user interface (GUI) —The GUI, which allows users to interact with devices through the use of images, such as icons, rather than text, must be tested to ensure it meets specifications. This is done by developing test cases that use all the functions of the GUI. GUIs usually have a large number of operations, so size and sequencing of actions are important considerations. Open source and commercial testing applications are available for GUI testing.

Installation—This tests the procedures needed to install, uninstall, and upgrade applications. All configurations should be tested, including installing on various types of equipment.

Maintenance—This testing is done to identify problems requiring maintenance with equipment or applications or to evaluate the effectiveness of repairs. Maintenance testing is often done on software already in use when it is changed in some way or installed in other hardware.

Recovery—This involves purposely crashing the system and evaluating the system's ability to recover. Techniques include restarting the computer in the middle of an action, unplugging the device during data retrieval, and restarting a browser after accessing a number of different windows to determine if memory and access to the windows remain intact after restarting.

Regression—This tests the system after a change, such as installation of a patch or a change in configuration, to determine if the change has introduced faults into the system.

Sanity—This is rapid run-through testing to determine if results seem reasonable and the system appears to work correctly. This type of testing may be done during development and before more rigorous testing to find obvious faults.

Scalability—This tests the ability of the system to function under increasing loads (scaling up) or under increasing nodes (scaling out), such as adding computers or servers to the system. Scaling may be strong or weak.

Security—This testing is done to determine if data security is adequate in protecting confidentiality. It also tests authentications, access controls, availability of information, and nonrepudiation (ensuring a record remains of messages sent and received). Steps include discovery, scanning for vulnerability, assessing vulnerability, assessing security, conducting penetration tests to simulate an attack on the system, auditing, and reviewing.

Smoke/power on—This involves attaching an electronic device to power and observing the result ("smoke"). This identifies overloads or overheating. In computer applications, this refers to initial testing to identify failures ("smoke"). Smoke tests may be functional (testing the entire program) or unit (testing specific functions).

Software performance—These tests are used to determine the ability of the system to perform under specified workloads. Software performance testing may include load testing, stress testing to determine upper limits, endurance testing to determine the length of time a system can function under an anticipated load, spike testing to determine if the system can function with a sudden dramatic increase in load, configuration testing to determine if the system functions with changes in configuration, and isolation testing to repeat tests that resulted in failures or system problems.

Usability—This tests the ability of end-users to use the system and applications adequately. This may involve observation and "think aloud" to evaluate performance, accuracy, ability to recall steps, duration of time spent on tasks, and personal response.

System Maintenance

System maintenance activities encompass both the hardware and software aspects of keeping the system "caught up" in terms of maintenance. Hardware activities revolve around the consumables and physical storage requirements associated with printing and backing up system data. Software activities are associated with the updates of system software and the related testing/change control procedures. Specific system maintenance tasks include:

- Troubleshooting hardware and software problems.
- Keeping an adequate supply of replacement hardware (e.g., printers, cables, and monitors) and consumables (e.g., toner and ink cartridges).
- Performing system back up procedures according to a predefined schedule.
- Making sure the system has enough storage capacity.
- Applying system upgrades and software patches.
- Making sure disaster recovery plan is in place and ready for implementation.

Common Problems Seen When Managing System Issues

During the implementation stage of a new system and conversion of data, a number of **common problems** may occur, including the following:

- Inadequate allocation of time and resources needed to implement a new system.
- Frequent changes that require programming revisions and result in both scope creep and feature creep with added costs in terms of time and finances.
- Underestimation of the amount of customization required to implement a system and convert data. (One solution is to resist all customization and another, to fully customize.)
- Failure to budget or plan for service contracts, updates, technical support, power needs, and ongoing operating costs.
- Inadequate testing of all components and the system, resulting in problems with conversion.
- Failure to understand the need for training and inadequate resource allocation for training and training materials.
- Failure to assess user resistance accurately or build support for system changes.

Requirements of System Issues Management

A number of different criteria must be considered for effective **system issues management**:

- **Technical:** Type of architecture, downtime necessary for maintenance, standards for connectivity, environments for testing, response times, and supporting technologies.
- **General/managerial:** Security standards, data standards, options for storage, capabilities related to providing reports, integration with health information exchanges.
- **Registration:** Correct client identification with unique identifiers across multiple registration sites and ability to track client's location and use of services.
- **Computerized physician order entry reporting:** Indicates details about orders, provides notification of duplicate orders, produces audit trail, supports documentation, generates claims, provides clinical decision support, and displays results.
- **Integrated documentation:** Pulls documentation (e.g., claims) from various departments.
- **Scheduling:** Appointments, testing, and procedures.
- **Medical records:** Provides automatic coding.
- **Billing:** Provides summaries, insurance information, and charges.

System Failure

System failure may result in the hardware freezing or software malfunctioning. In some cases, the system may reboot, but in other cases, it may simply stop functioning. Error messages may help to indicate the type of problem that is occurring and may guide troubleshooting efforts. Policies should be in place to guide procedures during the time the system is not available (e.g., downtime planning). Common causes of system failure include user/operator error, power disruptions/disconnections, overheating, and equipment malfunction or failure. Fast response to identify the cause of the system failure and repair to get the system up and running again are essential, but recovery, such as entering paper-stored data, must also be completed along with verification to ensure that data have not been corrupted and that the system is functioning properly.

User Experience

Human–Computer Interaction Framework

The **human–computer interaction (HCI) framework** developed by **Nancy Staggers** in 2001, applies concepts related to psychology and technology to explain human interactions with computers over a period of time in different contexts. The different contexts include the following:

- Providers
- Patients
- Interactions between patients and providers

Communication is the basic exchange of human–computer interactions. The basic tasks to accomplish this exchange include initiating interaction, responding, providing information, and exchanging information. The primary focus of HCI is usability related to human performance during interactions with computers in different contexts, such as overall ease of use, difficulty in learning, efficiency, satisfaction, the ability to carry out error-free interactions, and the ability of the computer system to match the tasks. Another focus is the mental model of users, the idea that the response of users to computers is based on previous knowledge and experience. In order to be successful in tackling complex computer tasks, the mental model should be consistent with the concept or design of the computer programs; thus, the goal is to find a design that promotes an effective mental model.

Software Usability

A key factor in **choosing software** for a computer system is the software's usability. Overall, usability is based on "user-centric" design that incorporates the interaction of the human user from the start of the design process. The success (or failure) of the design is based upon measurements such as focus groups, interviews, or questionnaires with the targeted potential users of the software. For software developers, it is important to remember to balance usability with utility. The software must be able to collect the proper inputs and perform its primary designed function in addition to having the best possible human interface (in terms of usability). Once the software is installed, the targeted users should also test it for usability. This should include a variety of individuals from all areas of the organization. The data collected should then be shared with the software developer for usability enhancements in future versions.

There are three different factors that contribute to software usability. They are:

- **Learnability:** The amount of time it takes to learn and figure out how to use the software program. This can be enhanced by the program's help features, documentation, and interface design.
- **Memorability (or efficiency):** The amount of time it takes the user to perform tasks without having to stop and look up the instructions or use the help feature. Software that has been intuitively designed will enhance memorability.
- **Discovery:** The time it takes a user to find specific product features in response to the need for that particular feature. This may be enhanced by the similarity of a software product to one that was previously used.

All three of these factors should be evaluated when determining whether to purchase a software program for an information system.

Usability or Ease of Use

An important aspect of human–computer interaction (HCI) is **usability** or **ease of use**, which may encompass a variety of elements, such as screen layout and navigation. The three primary goals of usability are effectiveness, efficiency, and satisfaction. Usability studies should address all of these goals. There are many different approaches to usability studies, but studies have indicated that large-scale studies can often be replaced with small-scale studies with five to eight participants. Practice with prototypes, even on paper, can yield valuable insights. Participants using the prototypes are encouraged to "think aloud" and talk through the procedures, while observers write down the observations. This can help to determine the ease of use of equipment or software and the amount of training needed for effective use. Evaluation by trained experts can also effectively highlight usability problems. Heuristic (rule of thumb) evaluation or inspection methods have been developed to help guide the evaluation process. Measures of user perceptions include asking participants to assign usability ratings, noting comments during use, and administering questionnaires about satisfaction and workload.

Conducting Usability Studies

These are the **steps for conducting a usability study**:
1. **Defining Purpose** - The purpose, which guides the choice of usability tests, should be clearly defined.
2. **Evaluating constraints** - The constraints (e.g., time, staff, resources) may influence the type of testing and the design of the test.
3. **Refining components based on evaluation of human–computer interaction (HCI) framework** - The HCI framework must be evaluated to determine each component and to whom or what it applies. This includes choosing the most appropriate staff, determining the most important step in a process, and choosing the setting. If testing involves comparison with older or more traditional practices, then measures of equivalency must be determined.
4. **Determining emphasis** - Usability testing may focus on one or more aspects, depending on the overall purpose.
5. **Select methods** - Methods must match purpose and take into account constraints and HCI evaluation.

Performance Testing to Assess for Errors

Performance testing to **assess for errors** includes the following:
- Time needed to complete tasks, including both the speed and reaction time.
- Percentage of completed and incomplete tasks and the percentage completed correctly.
- Number of errors and types of errors.
- Time spent in each component/option as well as frequency.
- Time spent in training.
- Overall quality of completed tests.
- Time needed for system setup or installation and ease or complexity.
- Users descriptions of problems encountered and "think aloud" comment during tasks.
- Degree of application usage in real work environment as opposed to testing.
- Observations of user responses and behavior, including facial expressions, actions, and eye tracking.
- Amount of time spent on the internet and the number of hits.

Assessing Types of Errors

When performing modeling studies to determine the **number of errors** that occur in human–computer interactions, the **types of errors** should also be considered. With input, errors may occur during intention to carry out actions, the sequence, or the execution. With output, errors may occur in perception, interpretation, or evaluation:

- **Low level:** Errors in execution of steps interfere with outcomes, and misunderstanding of outcomes interferes with perception.
- **Moderate level:** The sequence of actions results in input that is not compatible with the computer or the mode results in misinterpretation of input. Output is misunderstood or misinterpreted because of a lack of training or education.
- **High level:** Interference with intention occurs because of an inability to make a decision regarding a correct action or an inability to evaluate and interpret outcomes correctly.

Cognitive Walkthrough and Ease of Learning

Cognitive walkthrough is one method to determine **ease of learning** of new technology or applications. A study to determine each step in a process to complete a task is completed. Cognitive walkthrough is one method to assess the user's ability to understand the model and its purpose, to produce the desired actions, and to determine if users understand which is the right action and system feedback. The "think aloud" procedure is used while participants use a product and carry out the steps in a process, noting any usability problems, such as the ability to learn the process without formal training. Sessions may be audiotaped or videotaped for later evaluation. Cognitive walkthroughs are particularly useful with prototypes or early in a system to identify problems with design or usability. Users may also be assessed for knowledge retention over a period of time and their comprehension of the system.

Software Likeability and Utility

Likeability of software programs is not the same as usability or utility. Usability is the ease of which a human uses a software program. Likeability is defined as how much an individual enjoys using the program. Products that rank high in usability tend to also get high marks for likeability. While it is difficult to pinpoint exactly why users prefer one software program to another, likeability is a leading factor in determining how much a person wants to use the software.

Utility is the usefulness of the program. Utility does play a role in the likeability of a product. If the user perceives that the software will perform correctly, they are more likely to use it. They may also be attracted to the cost saving potential of the software program.
Both of these factors should be considered when purchasing system software.

Supporting End-Users

System Support

The role of **system support** encompasses all of the activities required to make sure the system is operating as it was designed to perform. Performance issues (e.g., a slow system response time) may indicate that the system is about to crash. Detection of problems is as important as troubleshooting items that have already broken. Specific system support activities include:
- Fielding all requests made during the implementation period.
- Establish ongoing communication between the system administrators and the system users. This may take the form of a printed newsletter, e-mail updates, or an in-house focus group.
- Establishing a 24-hour telephone help desk.
- Performing follow-up to all completed help requests to verify that the problem was adequately resolved.

Creation of Standard Operating Procedures (SOPs) and User Manuals

The following steps should be followed when developing the **documentation** that will be used to operate the new information system:
- **Step 1:** The standard operating procedures and user documentation should be prepared and used to train users before the system goes live.
- **Step 2:** The documentation that was used to operate the old system should be evaluated for applicability (via editing) to operate the new system.
- **Step 3:** Disaster recovery documents should be prepared in the event the system "crashes" or goes down. A paper-based system should be readily available.
- **Step 4:** The vendor's user guides and support documentation should be reviewed to determine if the information could be incorporated in the organization's user documentation.

End-User Acceptance and User-Acceptance Testing

Analysis of **end-user acceptance** of systems using human–computer interactions or **user-acceptance testing (UAT)** is done to determine the end-users willingness to use computer technology and software in the way in which it is designed. Without acceptance, users may avoid or misuse technology or remain dissatisfied, impacting job performance. For successful implementation of a system, user acceptance is critical. Analysis of end-user acceptance should begin during alpha (completed by developer) or beta (completed by end-users) testing before complete implementation of a system. Usability testing should help to determine ease of use and inherent problems in the system. While some organizations use surrogate end-users for testing, at least some participants should be actual end-users. Steps to analyzing end-user acceptance include:
- Analyzing the basic requirements of the system and the organization.
- Identifying the end-user acceptance scenarios.
- Describing a testing plan, including different severity levels based on real-world conditions.
- Designing the testing plan and test cases, considering the risks and the skills of the end-users.
- Conducting the tests.
- Evaluating and recording results.

Help-Desk Ticket System

The informatics nurse should routinely assess **help-desk tickets** to determine the types of problems that end-users are encountering. Whether the organization utilizes an automated cloud-based hosted service or an inhouse service, the help desk should maintain records of all calls or requests, so the informatics nurse can review the tickets and assess whether problems are scattered or if a pattern, such as increased types of one request or increased requests from one unit, emerges. Having a standardized help-desk request form, which can be filled in online, is especially useful to track issues. Any time there is an increase in requests, the informatics nurse should evaluate the types of requests (looking for patterns), interview the help-desk staff for their input, and interview and observe end-users. Based on these assessments and observations, the informatics nurse may recommend changes in hardware, software programming, or additional training for end-users.

Product Analysis

Product analysis may be used to analyze one product or to compare a number of products. Product analysis may be conducted during the design of a product at any stage but may also be conducted to determine if existing products or prototypes meet desired criteria. Product analysis focuses on how products are made and used and their important features. Product analysis helps to identify flaws or problem areas in a product and can identify possible changes needed for improvement. Steps in product analysis include:
- Selecting product or products to be analyzed.
- Determining the target market or user.
- Establishing a list of criteria: cost, usability, user learning curve, user satisfaction, integration, product construction and materials, quality, dimensions, safety, life cycle, and recyclability.
- Determining a scoring or ranking scale (e.g., 1 to 5, good to bad).
- Evaluating the products in terms of each criterion and assigning a score or rank.
- Assessing scores or ranks for problems or flaws.
- Identifying changes needed in product.

Market Analysis

Market analysis is done to determine both the current status of the market for a product or service and the future potential. Market analysis includes assessment of the following:
- **Size of the market and demand:** Current data about sales from government, industry, surveys, and major producers of similar products or services.
- **Marketing trends:** Regulations, social factors, environmental factors, innovations, and any factors that may affect sales.
- **Growth rate of market:** Based on analysis of historical data, current sales data, and developments that may impact growth positively or negatively.
- **Opportunity assessment:** In terms of competition.
- **Profitability:** Assessment of influencing factors (Michael E. Porter), including buyer and supplier power, barriers to market entry, possible threat of competitive substitute products or services, and company rivalry.
- **Cost structure:** Determining value and costs.
- **Methods of distribution:** Existing and emerging.
- **Necessary factors:** Resources, access to distribution, and technology.

Analyzing End-User Acceptance of Systems

The primary purpose of most end-user testing is to identify errors. Testing may be done to verify that the system functions as intended or to validate that the system functions in a way that meets the requirement of an organization. A number of different methods can be used to **analyze end-user acceptance** of systems.

- User acceptance testing with scenarios in which users carry out representative tasks.
- Interviews with users regarding usability and other problems.
- Questionnaires for users to determine perceptions of usability.
- Comparative studies with users using different systems or methods.
- Direct observation of users carrying out tasks.
- Indirect observation of users carrying out tasks, such as by video.
- Analysis of computer-generated data to determine accuracy and numbers of errors.

Reporting an Analysis to Stakeholders

When **reporting an analysis to stakeholders**, the first step is to determine the factors that are most important to the specific stakeholders. For example, management may be most interested in cost-effectiveness while end-users may be most interested in ease of use. Thus, the report should focus on the areas of interest. While analysis may have involved many steps, a report is most concerned with the end result of the analysis: "This is what works" rather than "This is how we know what works." Data should be presented in a visual medium, such as in charts or diagrams, as much as possible so stakeholders can more easily comprehend. PowerPoint presentations may be used but should contain supporting charts or highlights, not the entire report, as stakeholders will focus on the screen rather than the presenter. The report should be outlined in advance, organized in a meaningful way (most important information to least important, or vice versa), and presented clearly, allowing time for questions.

Adoption Surveys

When formulating an **adoption survey**, it's important to determine the type of information that is needed, and this may best be obtained through collaboration with end-users so that user needs are fully understood. A poorly designed survey may provide little valuable insight. For example, if a survey simply assesses acceptance of the new system and the results are negative, this alone does not help to determine where the problem lies and may, in fact, just reflect a common resistance to change. Surveys should be specific and may be targeted to specific groups of staff, so a number of surveys may be necessary to evaluate implementation. Once the surveys are completed, the results should be quantified and reviewed to determine if patterns emerge. These patterns, then, should be targeted for intervention through modifications in the system or additional training of staff members.

Performance Reports

Performance reports should provide quantifiable data to show how resources are being utilized to achieve system objectives. Performance reports require the collection of data as well as presentation, which may occur in many different formats. Two typical types of performance reports include:

- **Status reports:** These may be in various formats and may be automatically triggered, such as routine computerized reports, or completed by individuals, such as narrative reports that describe processes or the duration needed to carry out certain tasks and current costs.
- **Progress reports:** These list tasks accomplished during a specific period of time, such as weekly or monthly. Progress reports are especially important during implementation.

Performance reports may be provided in periodic status review meetings that allow for better exchange of information. All performance reports should be reviewed carefully to determine what is performing well and what requires modification.

Data Management and Health Care Technology

Data Standards

Metadata and Semantic Representation

Metadata is data that are used to describe other data. For example, if a hospital website contains a photograph, the metadata may provide information about resolution, date the photograph was taken, and the name of the photographer. Websites often have meta tags (HTML codes) that lead to stored information that is not displayed, such as key words and additional information. Metadata is often accessed by search engines to determine which files to access.

Semantic representation refers to the fact that terms in a system must have a standardized meaning and should be unambiguous. That is, a term represents meaning that must be understood the same way throughout the system and be part of the vocabulary utilized so that, for example, when accessing information about "falls," the term must be clearly understood in terms of what a fall represents. Semantic representation is important to consider when designing systems because it is necessary to adequately access data.

Electronic Health Record (EHR)

The **Healthcare Information and Management Systems Society (HIMSS)** define the **electronic health record (EHR)** as a "secure, real-time, point-of-care, patient-centric information resource for clinicians."

HIMSS has also published a series of guidelines for EHR known as the HIMSS Electronic Health Record Definitional Model. According to the model, the EHR should record and manage information for both the short- and long-term. The EHR should be the healthcare professional's main resource when taking care of patients. Evidence-based care can be planned using the EHR on both the individual and community level. Another important job of the EHR is its use in continuous quality improvement, performance management, risk management, utilization review, and resource planning. The EHR aids in the billing process as well. Finally, the EHR is a boon to evidence-based research, clinical research, and public health reporting. Since it is computerized, clinicians are assured that the EHR information is up to date and relevant for patients and research protocols.

Health Information Exchanges and Regional Health Information Organizations

Health information exchanges (HIEs) have been developed to allow exchange of health information among different health care providers in a specified area, region, or system. Information is shared electronically, saving costs and speeding access. Health Information Technology for Economic and Clinical Health included grants through the National Coordinator of Health Information Technology for the establishment of organizations, known as **regional health information organizations (RHIOs)**, to facilitate HIEs. According to federal guidelines, an RHIO is a neutral organization that complies with the structure of participating organizations. RHIOs vary in structure, but basic functions include facilitating connectivity that allows data to be effectively and securely exchanged across local, regional, or state HIEs. RHIOs provide management services and oversight of HIEs. Other services provided by RHIOs include: improved patient care, avoidance of service duplication, improved administrative efficiency, integration of preventive care, improved response times, facilitated interchanges with public health departments, and education.

Regional Health Improvement Plans

Regional health improvement plans (RHIPs) are developed to improve the delivery of health care. RHIPs cover all aspects of health care, including risk factors, diagnosis, treatment, disability, and social/mental factors, as well as all delivery systems, including hospitals, clinics, and individual practitioners. RHIPs establish prioritized strategic goals, such as improving health care while reducing costs as well as research and protocols needed to achieve these goals. Some RHIPs are regional while others, such as Oregon's RHIP, are statewide initiatives. Elements usually included in RHIPs are adherence to federal guidelines, policies, design of system, outcome measures, quality improvement methods to integrate services, and education and workforce development. Statewide RHIPs or those encompassing a large region may contain many subplans focused on particular areas of health care, such as mental health.

NANDA-I, Nursing Interventions Classification, and Nursing Outcomes Classification

Outlined below are three classification systems used in nursing informatics:
- **NANDA-I** (North American Diagnosis Association-International)
  - There are 167 classified diagnoses defined and characterized in this system.
- **Nursing Interventions Classification (NIC)**
  - There are 514 treatments performed by nurses.
  - System also provides links to NANDA diagnoses.
  - System is categorized into 44 specialty practice areas.
- **Nursing Outcomes Classification (NOC)**
  - Provides expected outcomes for patients, caregivers, family members, and community members for 330 disease states.
  - System includes definitions, indicators, measurement tools, and references.

Using these in designing information systems ensures that terms and conditions follow established standards that can be compared across a wide swath of healthcare organizations. Consistent information is also helpful when publishing results.

Perioperative Nursing Data Set, SNOMED CT, and the Patient Care Data Set

Outlined below are the Perioperative Nursing Data Set, SNOMED CT, and the Patient Care Data classification systems:
- **Perioperative Nursing Data Set (PNDS):** The perioperative nursing data set provides uniform terms for patient problems that may occur during an operation. It also provides terms for the related resources and observed outcomes.
  - Includes diagnostic and intervention components.
  - Provides documentation standards framework.
- **SNOMED CT (Systematized Nomenclature of Medicine Clinical Terms):** SNOMED CT is a comprehensive collection of clinical terms.
  - 357,000 concepts defined and categorized.
  - 957,000 descriptions.
  - Available in English, German, and Spanish.

- **Patient Care Data Set (PCDS):** The Patient Care Data Set is a data dictionary designed to provide a standard set of terms (capturing clinical data) for inclusion in healthcare information systems.
  - Developed by Dr. Judith Ozbolt.
  - Classification for problems, goals, and orders.

Clinical Care Classification and the Omaha System

Outlined below is the Clinical Care Classification system and the Omaha System used for data entry in the medical field:
- **Clinical Care Classification (CCC)**
  - This system was formerly known as Home Health Care Classification (HHCC).
  - The system uses two major subsets of information:
  - Diagnoses and outcomes: The terms used in the specific diagnosis and outcomes of a disease state.
  - Interventions and actions: For a given disease state, the appropriate interventions and actions.
  - There are 21 "Care Components" which classify care over a wide range of factors such as functional, physiological, and psychological.
- **Omaha System**
  - Uses a Problem Classification Scheme (assessment). This scheme allows for evaluating the condition of the patient.
  - Intervention Scheme. The intervention scheme prescribes the appropriate interventions to treat the problem (or disease state).
  - Problem Rating Scale for Outcomes (in terms of knowledge, behavior, and status). The scale ranges from 1 to 5 (a Likert type scale).

Logical Observation Identifiers Names and Codes, International Classification for Nursing Practice, and Nursing Management Minimum Data Set

Logical Observation Identifiers Names and Codes (LOINC): This database of terms is used primarily for laboratory results. By using uniform terms, the data can be grouped for analysis or transmitted to other computer systems.
- Begun for laboratory terms.
- 32,000 terms that include clinical information and codes for nursing observations.

International Classification for Nursing Practice (ICNP): The ICNP provides uniform terms for nursing data. Again, the goal is to create a system in which data can be examined and transmitted to other computers systems in a recognizable way.
- Sponsored by the International Council of Nurses.
- Categories for diagnosis, interventions, and outcomes.

Nursing Management Minimum Data Set (NMMDS): The NMMDS is a dynamic collection of standardized terms related to nursing. The goal is to create terms that will allow data to be compared across a wide swath of computer systems.
- Terminology for describing context and environment.
- Include categories for personnel characteristics, financial resources, and population data.

Current Procedural Terminology Codes

Current procedural terminology (CPT) codes were developed by the American Medical Association and used to define those licensed to provide services as well as medical and surgical treatments, diagnostics, and procedures. The CPT 2012 codes cover specific procedures as well as typical times required for treatment. The CPT codes are usually updated each October with revisions (additions, deletions) to coding. The use of CPT codes is mandated by both the Centers for Medicaid and Medicare and the Health Insurance Portability and Accountability Act (HIPAA) to provide a uniform language and to aid research. These codes are used primarily for billing purposes for insurance (public and private). Under HIPAA, Health and Human Services has designed CPT codes as part of the national standard for electronic health care transactions. Category I codes are used to identify a procedure or service. Category II codes are used to identify performance measures, including diagnostic procedures. Category III codes identify temporary codes for technology and data collection.

International Classification of Disease Codes

The **International Classification of Disease (ICD) codes**, developed by the World Health Organization to acquire worldwide morbidity and mortality data, are used to code for diagnoses. ICD-10 (2010) is the current version, and adoption was required by 2013 because version 10 contains codes to implement electronic health records (EHRs) and other electronic transactions. Version 11, which can be used with health information systems, is in development and will facilitate internet-based editing. This version will be released in 2018. ICD-9 diagnoses were used by all providers, but ICD-9 procedures were used only for inpatients; however, use is expanded with ICD-10, which is much more specific. ICD-10 contains twenty-two chapters with numerous subcategories; for example, Chapter I, "Certain Infectious and Parasitic Diseases"(A00–B99) lists inclusions, exclusions, and twenty-one subcategories, such as viral hepatitis (B15–B19). These subcategories have further divisions; for example, viral hepatitis B15 includes hepatitis with hepatic coma (B15-0) and without (B15-09). An electronic training tool is available on the internet. ICD-10 is consistent with the *Diagnostic and Statistical Manual of Mental Disorders*, 5th edition; cancer registry codes; and nursing classifications.

Clinical Context Object Workgroup

Clinical Context Object Workgroup (CCOW) is an HL7 workgroup that develops standard protocols for the sharing of information among applications at the point of care through context management. For example, data about a patient may be contained in a number of different applications and locations, but the CCOW allows a user to sign in one time and do one search (e.g., for a patient) for simultaneous access to information found in all the applications. CCOW may be used for internet-based on non-internet-based access. CCOW defines the standards that allow interoperability and focuses on the use of technology neutral architecture and widely used computer technology. CCOW works in collaboration with the HL7 Security Workgroup to ensure protection of data. The CCOW does not do specific designs or implementation but aims to provide standards to facilitate implementation and effective design. CCOW allows both internet (http) and Active X (a Microsoft software) mapping.

International Organization for Standardization

The **International Organization for Standardization (ISO)**, a nongovernmental organization, encompasses a network of standard institutes, public and private, in 164 countries and develops and publishes voluntary international standards based on consensus. The standard institutes are the primary bodies approving standards for the countries they represent. Standards for government, business, and society are developed in partnership with end-users, ensuring that those using the standards have input. The ISO currently has over 19,500 international standards for a wide range of sectors, including health care, management, and organizational practice, although the ISO does not provide certification or accreditation. The ISO is also involved in conformity assessment to ascertain if standards are followed. The ISO has established partnerships with numerous organizations, such as the World Trade Organization, and collaborates with the United Nations. Additionally, the ISO has established a code of ethics that includes a commitment to meeting future needs, development of international standards in a fair and responsive manner, promoting implementation, monitoring, and protecting the image and integrity of the ISO, and helping developing countries.

Standards in Information Storage, Creation, Analysis, and Retrieval

The **National Institutes of Health** (NIH) is working toward implementing **standards** in the area of medical informatics. They recently began a push for standards in information storage, creation, analysis, and retrieval (ISCAR). Huge amounts of medical data are being created every year. In order for this information to be compiled effectively, international standards are necessary. The creation of interoperational databases is essential. There is far too much information produced each year to fit into a single database. As an example, one research laboratory can produce enough information to fill one million encyclopedias in the course of one year's work. In addition, key to this process is the importance of software that can analyze data taken from different databases. The rationale for this whole scheme is to allow for more comparative studies, make peer review simpler, and lend ease to verification of results.

Industry Standards Associated with Nursing Informatics

There are two major **standards** associated with nursing informatics:
- The Institute of Electrical and Electronic Engineers (IEEE) developed the P1073 Medical Information Bus (MIB) standards to aid in the transfer of information between patient medical devices and the hospital's mainframe computer system. Patient medical devices are updated in real-time as they are used in emergency rooms, intensive care units, and operating rooms. These standards are built into all such devices universally to avoid problems with data communication. The latest series of standards, 802.11 also known as Wi-Fi, allow for computers and medical devices to communicate wirelessly.
- The National Electrical Manufacturers Association and the American College of Radiologists created Digital Imaging and Communications in Medicine (DICOM). Digital Imaging and Communications in Medicine is used in association with biomedical images and image-related information. While not the only standard of its kind, it is the primary one used in North America.

American Society for Testing and Materials

One of the largest standards development organizations is **the American Society for Testing and Materials (ASTM).** The role of the ASTM is to create standard methods for testing materials and procedural testing standards for different industries. For computing, the ASTM has established standards for content and verification of different computer protocols. The ASTM has developed over 9,000 standards in a wide range of fields. However, the E1384-96, E1633-95, and E31 are of primary importance to the healthcare industry. E1384-96 was developed by ASTM in 1996 and gives information on how to set computer-based patient record (CPR) content. E1633-95 was developed in 1995 and set the definition for coded values within a CPR. There are currently about 30 standards developed by ASTM by committee E31 that specify the information necessary for a patient's continuity of care record (CCR) and how that information should be presented in an electronic format, and many more standards are still in the process of being drafted.

Health Level 7 (HL7) and Fast Healthcare Interoperability Resources (FHIR)

Health Level 7 (HL7) is an international standard developing organization that sets standards used in the sharing, retrieval, exchange, and integration of electronic health information (clinical and administrative) among different healthcare computer systems. In 2007, HL7 developed standards regarding functions needed in an EHR: direct care, supportive (administrative, financial), and information infrastructure (interoperability, security, workflow). HL7 is accredited by the American National Standards Institute (ANSI) and is committed to ensuring interoperability of health care information management systems (HIMS). There are seven categories of standards: primary, foundational, clinical and administrative domains, EHR profiles, implementation guides, rule and references, and education and awareness. HL7 created the **fast healthcare interoperability resources (FHIR),** which is a standard for data formats and a web-based application programming interface (API) to facilitate the exchange of EHRs among healthcare providers. FHIR allows healthcare organizations to collect real-time data.

Data Management

Data management in healthcare refers to the use of computers to store, access, and secure patient information. Personnel who are responsible for data management include those who input the information, system analysts, programmers, and database administrators. Information may be stored as tables in a relational database. Some organizations may connect to data warehouses in order to access very large amounts of stored information. Data warehouses are often used to store results from clinical trials or insurance membership information. Many healthcare organizations have stopped using paper documents all together because of the cost required to store and retrieve paper files. Paper documents are also more susceptible to physical damage and loss than computerized data. Some companies have scanned paper documents into their new computer systems through a process known as document imaging. Additionally, some facilities use document imaging to transfer patient test results (e.g., radiological film) into their computerized record system.

Data Warehouse

An organization's past computerized information is kept in a data warehouse. This is the information that is not required on a daily basis by the typical system user, but is used by management to make decisions. It is important that a data warehouse be configured so that a data analyst can research information quickly and effectively. An effective data warehouse as has the following characteristics:

- **Subject-oriented:** This refers to the fact that all events or objects that are the same are linked in a traceable manner.
- **Time-variant:** This is the ability to look at how information changes as a function of time.
- **Non-volatile:** This means that once information is recorded, it can never be deleted or manipulated in a manner that could cause its loss.
- **Integrated:** This refers to the fact that information from all areas of the enterprise is placed into the same database for the sake of analysis.

There are **three major parts of a data warehouse**:

- **Infrastructure:** The infrastructure (sometimes referred to as the technology perspective) refers to the hardware and software used in the system.
- **Data:** Data are diagram representations of the structures that send and store information and how they relate to one another.
- **Process:** Process is defined by how information gets from one place to another or how it is dealt with.

Most data warehouses use the Codd rules of normalization, which breaks data down into a table in order to show the relationships between the various parts. Two widely used designs are:

- **Dimensional:** The dimensional approach breaks data down into numerical facts and reference information. Dimensionally based databases are easy to use and operate quickly. However, their structures are difficult to modify.
- **Normalized:** The normalized approach saves information in the "third normal form" and groups the information into tables according to their subjects. These databases can be slow and difficult to use.

Data warehouses were created as separate entities from ordinary computer system structures beginning in the late 1980s. The major reason for this type of setup was that separating the two functions freed up space and improved response time on the system servers. This structure also allowed for a centralized warehouse that could be used to create reports for the entire organization. There are **four types of data warehouses** that have evolved:

- **Offline operation databases:** Offline operational databases are simply copies of the operation system saved to a separate location or partition on the server.
- **Offline data warehouse:** The offline data warehouse creates a regular copy of the operational system used in a report-orientated system.
- **Real-time data warehouse:** Real-time data warehouses are similar to offline data warehouses except that they are constantly updated.
- **Integrated data warehouse:** An integrated data warehouse is updated with information, processes it, and returns the results to the central system for use in daily activities.

Medical/Clinical, Knowledge-Based, Comparison, and Aggregate Data

There are basically four types of **health care–related data**:

- **Medical/clinical data:** This information is patient-specific and includes information regarding the patient, diagnosis, treatment, laboratory findings, consultations, care plans, physician orders, informed consent, and advance directives. The medical record includes all procedures, discharge summary, and emergency care.
- **Knowledge-based data:** This information includes methods to ensure that staff is provided training, support, research, library services or other access to information, and good practice guidelines.
- **Comparison data:** These data may relate to internal comparisons or external comparisons to benchmarks or best-practice guidelines.
- **Aggregate data:** These data include pharmacy transactions, required reports, demographic information, financial information, hazard and safety practices, and any data not included in the clinical record.

Qualitative, Quantitative, Primary, and Secondary Data

Both qualitative and quantitative data are used for analysis, but the focus is quite different:

- **Qualitative data**—Data are described verbally or graphically, and the results are subjective, depending on observers to provide information. Interviews may be used as a tool to gather information, and the researcher's interpretation of data is important. Gathering these data can be time-intensive and usually cannot be generalized to a large population. This information gathering is often useful at the beginning of the design process for data collection.
- **Quantitative data**—Data are described in terms of numbers within a statistical format. This information gathering is done after the design of data collection is outlined, usually in later stages. Tools may include surveys, questionnaires, or other methods of obtaining numerical data. The researcher's role is objective.
- **Primary data**—Original data are collected for a particular purpose.
- **Secondary data**—Data were originally collected for another purpose.

Preserving Data Integrity

There are several common methods that **preserve data integrity**:

- **Staff education:** Employees who receive training on the documented correct use of the information system will be better equipped to enter and access information and determine that the information is correct.
- **System checks:** System error checks are written into computer programs so users are less likely to enter incorrect or inappropriate information (or omit mandatory information).
- **Data verification:** Data verification involves asking the patient to look over their information and verify whether it is correct or not. This process may be done in one of three ways. First, a staff member may read back the information to the patient and ask for a verbal confirmation. Second, the staff member may ask the patient to read and verify the information off the computer screen, continuing only once the data is verified. Third, the information may be printed onto paper with the patient reading it and formally signing a statement that it is correct.
- **Minimization of fraudulent information:** Establishing controls (such as checking a photo ID) to assure that the information entered is from the correct individual.

Attributes Used in Conceptual Data Models

Attributes are assigned to data that an organization collects. There are two important pieces of information that must be assigned to attributes:

- **Name:** The name of an attribute should be a one- or two-word definition. This enables the user to quickly realize what information is needed for that particular attribute. Examples used in healthcare are gender, physician's name, or date of birth. If possible, abbreviations should not be used as this can become confusing to the software programmer and user.
- **Domain:** The domain is the actual value an attribute can have. The attribute "gender" must be either male or female and "date of birth" must be a date. Domain information should have a defined format. For example, date of birth should always be entered as day/month/year with the year containing four digits. Defining domain formats allows the information entered by different users to be compared.

Discrete Data

Discrete data, usually used to represent the count of something, are those that have a specific value and cannot be further quantified. Because the person creating the database and the person providing data are often different, eliciting the correct discrete data can pose problems, especially if the person providing data is not well versed in database design. One of the first steps to ensuring adequate data is to do a requirement analysis, which involves eliciting information through case studies, interviews, focus groups, and observations. Identifying the types of data and interactions with the data is necessary to help determine what data are needed because data input must result in desired output.

Physical Database Design

A **physical database design** describes how information is accumulated, stored, accessed, and linked within the information system. In designing the system, it is important to know how it will be used. There are three factors to consider:
- **Queries** – The amount of data queries that will be required at any given time for the system.
- **Updates** – The frequency of updates and their effect on the database functions.
- **Performance** – The system speed, capacity, and overall robustness.

The next step is to decide on the number and types of indexes (hash or tree) that should be created. It is best to create indexes that can be used for a number of queries. This will optimize both storage space and access time.

Eliminating Redundancy

Eliminating redundancy is essential so as not to inflate a database. The first step is to identify attributes that are identifiers and those that provide information; then the redundant identification attributes can be removed. Redundancy also occurs when the same field is present in more than one table, which can lead to anomalies and data corruption. Normalization is the procedure used to eliminate redundancy and problems and to ensure that information is available from the database through querying. Large database tables are typically broken into smaller tables where redundancy is reduced and the relationship among the various tables is defined. Modifications (including insertions and deletions) in data should occur in one table rather than multiple tables.

Hierarchical and Relational Databases

Databases are computerized file structures that contain organized and accessible stored data. **Hierarchical databases**, the earliest type, are organized in a tree or parent–child formation with one piece of information connected to many (one-to-many), but in descending order only (not many-to-one). Hierarchical databases are appropriate only for simple structures (e.g., lists of e-mail addresses or telephone numbers) and have limited use in health care. Hierarchical databases have largely been replaced with **relational databases** (Edgar F. Codd, 1940), which are built on a multiple table structure with each individual item in a table having a unique identifier. The tables (or relationships) can be manipulated. Each table represents an item or thing. Tables are comprised of rows (i.e., records, which must be unique) and columns (i.e., fields). Relational databases allow both one-to-many and many-to-one relationships. Relational databases may contain over 1000 tables, but through querying, new tables, using the relationships among existing data, can be produced.

Decision Support Systems, Expert Systems, Artificial Intelligence Systems, and Natural Language Systems

Healthcare facilities may utilize a number of different systems:

Decision Support Systems
- Help people make judgments.
- Take all available data for a problem, generate results, implement the results in a simulation, and choose the optimum solution.
- Often used to make staffing decisions.

Expert Systems

- Similar to decision support systems, but using logic derived from specific task experts.
- Operate using "If, then" type logic drawing from a database of knowledge in the problem area.

Artificial Intelligence Systems

- Work using a model of human reasoning processes.
- Use the rules of inference such as "If A>B and B>C, then A must be greater than C."
- Attempt to find new ways to represent abstract ideas.
- Actually learn by trial and error.

Natural Language Systems

- Understand and process information in human language rather than programming language.
- Enable speech and handwriting recognition.

Management Information Systems, Bibliographic Retrieval Systems, Stand Alone Systems, Transaction Systems, and Physiologic Monitoring Systems

Management Information Systems (MIS): Strategic information technology (IT) planning that relates the capabilities of the organization to its customers and competitors. Includes the measured performance standards and the allocation of resources (for both human and technology needs). Includes operational support that provides information necessary for the day-to-day functioning of the organizational business units.

Bibliographic Retrieval Systems: Stores data for easy retrieval. As an example, MEDLINE is used to access journal articles and health information.

Stand Alone Systems: May also be called dedicated or turnkey systems. Used only for a specific function that does not require any connectivity.

Transaction Systems: Process specific transactions and produce reports that have the same format every time.

Physiologic Monitoring Systems: An input of electric impulses is converted to an output of waveforms. Examples: ECG, EEG, and the non-stress test.

Logging and Data Logging

Logging is an automatic process to record actions and events occurring in an information system in system log files, which contain a record of events for various components of the information system. Different systems have different log files, but they commonly provide information about devices, changes, and operations. Logs should be reviewed on a routine basis with reviews documented. Log files are used for auditing and are especially useful to evaluate applications, such as server applications, that have little end-user interaction. Log analysis software is available to assist in the evaluation of a log. **Data logging** allows the user to collect data, analyze, save, output results, and control the type of information collected, essentially as a method of computerized research. Data loggers are stand-alone devices that are used to acquire data, such as temperature and humidity in a server room.

Threats for Information Stored in Computerized Systems

The following are three **main threats for information** stored in computerized systems:
- **Quality** - Information quality may be compromised by the alteration of files. This may happen by accident (e.g., data corruption) or intentionally (e.g., forgery). There may also be an alteration of the system itself. This tends to happen during system upgrades or the introduction of unwanted programs (e.g., viruses, worms, or trojan horses).
- **Availability** - Availability of information may be threatened by power outages, damage to the system (or its parts), disaster or sabotage, or the system becoming overloaded.
- **Confidentiality** - Confidentiality may be compromised by personnel disobeying company policies (or procedures) or unauthorized individuals viewing printed records or computer screens.

Hazards Related to Storage on a Computer System

Though storing information on computer is considered safer than storing it on paper or microfilm, there are a number of **hazards** that should be taken into account and managed:
- **Environmental and Physical Safety:** This includes exposure to dust, extreme temperature, shock (e.g., earthquakes), humidity, water, and fire. Any one of these could compromise the integrity of computerized records.
- **Control:** This entails the physical and electronic access control mechanisms designed to protect the records from being erased, stolen, or altered.
- **Planning:** This is the process of creating backup copies of records and storing them in a separate location for safekeeping.
- **Time Restraints (Archiving):** This process determines how long information must be retained according to state and federal regulations and sets up a system for destruction of obsolete records.
- **Transfer:** These are plans to salvage records before they become unusable due to either degradation or changes in computer hardware.
- **Maintenance:** This includes upkeep of the system that writes and reads the data.

Disaster Recovery Plans

Disaster recovery plans are designed to make sure that the organization's operations can continue to function (at some level) throughout a disaster and return to full function once the disaster is over. Disaster recovery planning should be an ongoing process covering every conceivable scenario and involving all of the organization. It may be helpful to break a disaster recovery plan into modules (or sub-plans). Specific modules may include plans covering tests, maintenance, emergency, backup, and recovery. A test plan outlines ways that the organization can perform disaster recovery drills before they are actually needed. A maintenance plan outlines the steps needed to keep the whole disaster recovery plan up to date. An emergency plan is created to guide the organization during and right after a disaster. A backup plan lists all personnel who can be called in, alternate locations of data, and places that can be used to conduct business if the primary facility becomes unusable.

Many things can go **wrong with a disaster recovery plan** after a disaster. Unfortunately, many organizations fail to provide adequate support for operating under extreme situations. Some common areas that are sometimes found to be deficient include:

- **Documentation:** Critical documents should be stored in several locations (both digitally and in paper format).
- **Equipment:** As new equipment is purchased, it needs to be added to the plan.
- **Data storage:** Design the plan to allow quick recovery of critical information without needing to open an archive (or recover a database).
- **Keeping the plan updated:** Failing to keep the plan updated and failing to test the plan are two very common errors. Plans should be updated frequently and tested after each update.

Personal Health Records

Personal health records (PHRs) are electronic records that are generated by health care providers and the individual patient, allowing the patient to access, record, and share health information. Many different applications exist for creating a PHR. Elements of a PHR should include the following:

- The individual has the ability to control the PHR.
- The information in the PHR is comprehensive and covers the patient's lifetime.
- The information in the PHR derives from all health care providers.
- The PHR can be easily accessible at any time from any location with access.
- The information contained in the PHR is secure and cannot be accessed without proper authorization.
- The PHR discloses who enters data as well as who has accessed the data and when.
- Exchange of information with different health care providers across the health care system is efficient.
- PHRs should help to deliver care more cost-effectively and efficiently.

Paper/personal files: Patient-maintained paper records can include booklets, files, notebooks, medication records, and handwritten notations. While data can be aggregated from various sources, this method is time-consuming; quality varies widely, and data cannot always be easily retrieved.

Non-tethered: Nontethered PHRs are stand-alone and not connected to a particular system or electronic health record (HER). Information may be carried on a smart card, flash card, compact disc, or DVD. These pose more security risks than tethered PHRs and require more input from the individual to maintain accurate records.

Tethered: Data are tied to a particular system and EHR and are often internet-based. A secure patient portal is provided so the individual can access all or parts of the records, including lists of medications and laboratory results. Examples include Kaiser's HealthConnect and the Veterans Administration's My HealthVet. Interactivity varies but may include health diaries and logs.

Net-worked: Data are derived from multiple sources in a network rather than one system. This allows for more flexibility.

Basic principles for **networked personal health records (PHRs)** include:

- **Transparency:** Individuals should know the type of information that can be gathered about them, purpose, data location, who has access, and how individuals gain access.

- **Purpose:** The purpose of data collection should be provided when collected, and individuals should be apprised of change in purpose.
- **Consent limitations:** Individuals should consent to collection of information, and information should be limited to that necessary to fulfill the purpose of collection. Data should not be disclosed, distributed, or accessed for nonspecified purposes.
- **Control:** Individuals should control access to PHRs and know who stores information about them and for what purpose. They should also be able to review the method in which their information is used or stored.
- **Quality:** All information should be up-to-date and accurate.
- **Privacy and security:** Data should be safeguarded against unauthorized access, use, destruction, or alterations.
- **Oversight:** Those in control of data are responsible for implementing and maintaining principles.
- **Troubleshooting:** Methods must be readily available to address any breaches of security or privacy.

The **personal health record (PHR)** presents an opportunity for **patient use**, allowing patients to participate in their own health care in a number of ways:
- **Data entry:** Most PHRs allow patients to enter some types of data, although this varies. A typical data entry includes personal and family health history, use of complementary therapy, and health behaviors (e.g., diet, exercise). Some also allow entry of health data, such as blood pressure readings, daily blood sugar, and weight.
- **Delegation:** PHRs usually allow the patient to assign a delegate or proxy (e.g., caregiver, immediate family member) to access the PHR. In most systems, parents can access information for a child until age 13; the child may assign a parent as proxy after that age, although selected information (e.g., sexual history, treatment) may be blocked.
- **Messaging:** Many systems allow patients to send secure messages to health care providers, in some cases routing them through a triage team.

Querying from Databases

Data Retrieval

Information that has been stored in a computer system will eventually need to be accessed at some point. This process of accessing data is known as **data retrieval.** When choosing a system for data retrieval, the following factors are of importance:

- **Performance:** Performance should be measured by the time it takes for data to be retrieved and the number of requests that can be processed at one time.
- **Capacity:** Capacity refers to not just the number of files that can be stored, but also how large each file can be.
- **Data security:** Protecting the information from people who are not authorized to view it is a function of data security.
- **Cost:** There are three areas of concern involving cost: support personnel (those individuals who maintain the system), software (programs used for information retrieval), and hardware (the actual machines where the information is stored).

Boolean Logic

Boolean logic, developed by the mathematician George Boole in the 1800s, is used to search databases and is recognized by most search engines, such as Google. Search is conducted for keywords connected by the operators AND, OR, and NOT. Boolean searching is often used with truncations and wildcards:

- **Truncations:** "Finan*" provides all words that begin with those letters, such as "finance," "financial," and "financed."
- **Wildcards:** "m?n" or "m*n" provides "man" and "men."
- **AND:** "Wound AND antibiotic" produces all documents that contain both words.
- **OR:** "Wound OR Infect* OR ulcer" produces documents that contain "wound" and either "infect*" or "ulcer." This query is especially useful to search for a number of synonyms or variant spellings. This query may return a large number of documents. OR may be combined with other operators: Wound OR ulcer AND Povidone-iodine.
- **NOT:** Wound AND povidone-iodine NOT antibiotic NOT antimicrobial. NOT is used to exclude keywords.

Structured Query Language

The most common use of **structured query language (SQL)** is to obtain and display information from databases. SELECT is used with a number of optional keywords and extensions to access table data. The basic query includes SELECT, FROM (which columns and which table), WHERE, ORDER BY:

- Asterisk (*): shortcut to indicate all columns, such as SELECT*FROM customers
- Comma (,): used to list and separate specific columns, such as SELECT PatientID, LastName, FirstName, FROM County
- WHERE: limits the number of rows, such as SELECT PatientID, LastName, FirstNAME, From County = 'Monterey'
- NOT or <>: eliminates, such as FROM County <> 'Monterey'
- BETWEEN: limits, such as WHERE ServiceDate BETWEEN "1-july-2011' AND '1-September-2011'
- NOT IN: limits, such as WHERE City NOT IN ('Salinas', 'King City')

- LIKE: allows wild card characters _, %, [ ], [^]
- ORDER BY: dictates arrangement, such as SELECT PatientID, LastName, FirstName FROM County, ORDER BY County

Statistical Analysis System

Statistical Analysis System (SAS) is an integrated group of software applications used to report, analyze, and access data. Some applications are intended for programmers and others, for management. Statements and procedures are used to access functions. The three primary steps of an SAS program include the following:
- **Data**: uses SQL or FOCUS (a 4GL used to query databases) to automate identifying files
- **Procedures**: operate on the tables (data set) as a whole
- **Metaprogramming language**: metalanguage to write computer programs that affect other programs in some way (i.e., manipulate, reduce necessary code)

A number of different components are available, including the following:
- Base SAS software (SAS procedures, DATA debugger, output delivery system, windowing environment).
- Business intelligence dashboard: allows graphics that represent data.
- Data integration studio: extracts, transforms, and loads.
- Enterprise Business Intelligence services: collection of business tools.
- Enterprise miner: data mining tool.
- Information map studio: allows users to build information maps.

Data Analysis

Definitions Used in Data Analysis

Definitions used in data analysis must be based on a solid understanding of statistical analysis and epidemiological concepts. Specific issues that must be addressed include the following:
- **Sensitivity:** The data include all positive cases, taking into account variables and decreasing the number of false-negatives.
- **Specificity:** The data include only those cases specific to the needs of the measurement, excluding those from a different population thereby decreasing the number of false-positives.
- **Stratification:** Data are classified according to subsets, taking variables into consideration.
- **Recordability:** The tool/indicator collects and measures the necessary data.
- **Reliability:** Results should be reproducible.
- **Usability:** The tool or indicator should be easy to use and understand.
- **Validity:** Collection measures the target adequately, so that the results have predictive value.

Knowledge Discovery in Database and Data Mining

Knowledge discovery in database (KDD) is a method by which to identify patterns and relationships in large amounts of data, such as the identification of risk factors or the effectiveness of interventions. KDD may use data perturbation, the hiding of confidential information (e.g., names) while maintaining basic information in the database, and data mining. The steps to KDD include selecting data, preprocessing (e.g., assembling target data set, cleaning data of noise), transforming data, data mining, and interpreting results.

Data mining is the analysis (often automatic) of large amounts of data to identify underlying or hidden patterns. The effectiveness of data mining depends on many factors, such as hardware and software applications. Data mining may identify similar groupings in data, and these groups can then be further analyzed. Data mining may be applied to multiple patients' electronic health records to generate information about the need for further examination or interventions. The steps to data mining include detecting anomalies, identifying relationships, clustering, classifying, regressing, and summarizing.

Data mining involves electronically searching through large amounts of information to find relevant items. Data mining uses several tools to look for patterns:
- **Association rule mining:** This tool looks for patterns in which a certain data object shows up repeatedly (more than randomly) and is associated with an unrelated data object.
- **Classification:** This tool looks for data group membership. An example would be the number of sunny days in a year.
- **Clustering:** This tool organizes data objects according to their similar characteristics. This results in a natural pattern or clustering of similar data.

Data mining can also be called knowledge discovery. The results can also be used for making predictions. When drawing conclusions by use of mined data, statistical significance of relationships should be based on the sample size (with stricter rules for smaller data sets). Even though data mining has been in use for decades, there has been a recent public outcry against it (citing privacy concerns). Overall, data mining is a powerful tool that can be used for good purposes when used ethically.

Data Aggregation

Data aggregation refers to the collection and summation of data for further use, such as for statistical analysis. For example, data aggregation may be used to collect information about an individual from multiple sources, often for targeted marketing purposes. Most summary reports now contain aggregate data, but some data aggregation may be ineffective, impacting the results, so data aggregation must be planned and implemented accurately. Criteria include the following:

- Applications should integrate with existing hardware, software, and applications and should be adaptable and easy to manage.
- Applications should be flexible, using industry standards and supporting multiple reports.
- Performance should be fast, effective, and predictable.
- Results should be scalable.
- Implementation should be fast and efficient and require little training.
- Use of hardware and software should be efficient, requiring little increase in hardware, software, and storage.

Application should be cost-effective for the organization.

Measures of Averages

Measures of averages locate the center point of a group of data:

- **Mean** is the average number. However, since distribution can vary widely, the mean may not give an accurate picture. For example, if one unit has 20 infections per 100 and the other has 1 infection per 100, the mean $(21 \div 2)$ is 10.5 per 100, which has little validity.
- **Median** is the 50th percentile. For example, consider the following numbers: 1, 3, 7, 9, and 15. The number 7 is the median (middle) number. If there were an even number, the 2 middle numbers would be averaged: 1, 3, 7, 9, 14, and 15. The numbers 7 and 9 are averaged so the median is 8. If there is an even distribution, the mean and median will be the same. The wider the difference between the two, the more uneven the distribution.
- **Mode** is the number occurring with the highest frequency. There may be bimodal or trimodal numbers

Measures of Distribution

Measures of distribution show the spread or dispersion of data.

- **Range** is the distance from the highest to the lowest number. The term interquartile denotes the range between the 25th percentile and the 75th percentile. Range is usually reported with the median to provide information about both the center point and the dispersion.
- **Variance** measures the distribution spread around an average value. It is often used to calculate the effect of variables. A large variance suggests a wide distribution, and a small variance indicates that the random variables are close to the mean.

- **Standard deviation** is the square root of the variance and shows the dispersion of data above and below the mean in equally measured distances. In a normal distribution, 68% of the data are within 1 standard deviation (measured distance) of the mean, 95% of the data are within 2 standard deviations of the mean, and 99.7% of the data are within 3 standard deviations of the mean.

Chi-Square Test and *t* Test

Chi-square (X^2) is a method of comparing rates or ratios. The **chi-square test** is a means by which to establish if a variance in categorical data (as opposed to numerical data) is of statistical significance. There are a number of different approaches to chi-square testing, depending on the type of data, but it is generally used to show whether there is a significant difference between groups or conditions being analyzed. It may be used, for example, to compare the rates of surgical infections after two types of surgical procedures. The *t* **test** is used to analyze data to determine if there is a statistically significant difference in the means of both groups. The *t* test examines two sets of data that are similar, such as the average number of miles walked each week by women over 65 who have breast cancer as compared to women over 65 who do not have breast cancer.

Regression Analysis

Regression analysis is used to evaluate the data sets found in scattergrams; it compares the relationship between the dependent variable and the independent variable to determine if the relationship correlates. The strength of the relationship is indicated by the correlation coefficient (*r*), which ranges from 1 to + or − 1: −1 indicates a negative relationship in which one data set increases, and the other data set decreases; +1 indicates there is a positive relationship in which both data sets increase or decrease in which case the scattergram forms a straight line. The degree to which the data points form a straight line (strong correlation), loosely structured line (moderate correlation), or no line (no correlation) is reflected in the *r* value. An *r* value of 0 (midpoint) shows no relationship between the variables.

Integrating the Results of Data Analysis

Integrating the results of data analysis is necessary; attempting performance improvement and developing practice guidelines without data can be problematic. These data should be used not only as the basis for long-term strategic planning but also for identifying opportunities for performance-improvement activities on an ongoing basis. Integration of information includes:
- Identifying issues for tracking.
- Reviewing patterns and trends to determine how they impact care.
- Establishing action plans and desired outcomes based on the need for improvement.
- Providing information to process improvement teams to facilitate change.
- Evaluating systems and processes for follow-up.
- Monitoring specific cases, criteria, critical pathways, and outcomes.

The integration of information should assist with case management, decision-making about individual care, improvement of critical pathways related to clinical performance, staff performance evaluations, credentialing, and privileging.

Data Transformation

Data transformation is the process of changing information from a given source (such as a data entry terminal) into information that can be understood by a destination point (such as a large database). Data transformation is performed in two steps:

- **Data mapping.** This process develops a map of how information flows from one place to another and figures out which parts of the information needs to be transformed.
- **Code generation.** This is when the actual transformation occurs and the data is converted into a form compatible with its destination.

Following any transformation of data, it is important to conduct a test of data integrity. This confirmatory test will allow the user to check that no information was lost or incorrectly transformed during the process. Once a data transformation system has been created and proven sound, random tests for data integrity should still be performed on a regular basis.

Binary Code

Data representation can be verbal (e.g., spoken/written representations), analog (e.g., television, radio, telephone, recorded), or digital (e.g., coded). Analog representation uses continuous waveform signals varying in intensity. Computerized representation of data uses codes (usually numeric), such as the **binary code** (base 2) to represent values. The binary code is comprised of strings of 1s and 0s with 1s stored in magnetized areas of disks and 0s stored in nonmagnetized areas; thus, 1 represents "on," and 0 represents "off." Each representation (0 or 1) is referred to as a bit (binary digit). Data are converted into bits for digital transmission:

- 8 bits = 1 byte (can represent 256 characters).
- 1,000 bytes = 1 kilobyte.
- 1 million bytes = 1 megabyte.
- 1 billion bytes = 1 gigabyte.
- 1 trillion bytes = 1 terabyte.

The coding scheme is the pattern of 0s and 1s used to represent characters. For coding of English and European languages, the most common binary coding scheme is that of the American Standard Code for Information Interchange.

Hexadecimal Coding System

Because the binary system for representing decimal numbers results in much longer strings of digits, the **hexadecimal coding system** is often used. Hexadecimal characters represent 4 binary bits; thus, 1 byte can be represented by 2 hexadecimal characters. Hexadecimal coding uses a base of 16 and 16 symbols (usually the numeral 1–9, representing values 0 to 9 and Arabic letters A through F, representing values 10–15). One digit (4 bits) is referred to as a nibble, and 8 bits/1 byte are an octet. Additionally, coding may use # or &H in front of the code to indicate it is hexadecimal. For example, the number 10 is represented as #A. Binary code 1,000 is represented in hexadecimal code as 8. Conversion charts are available, so binary and hexadecimal coding can be easily converted from one to the other.

Unicode Standard Coding Scheme

The **unicode standard coding scheme**, used with the Universal Character Set, is a standardized coding system that has a large capacity and can be used to represent text for most languages, including Asian languages. Coding is available to represent technical characters, punctuation, and mathematic symbols. Unicode provides a specific numeric value for each character and can be used across multiple platforms. Unicode comprises approximately 110,000 characters, representing all alphabets of the world languages, ideographic sets, symbols, and 100 scripts, and is particularly valuable for making coding accessible internationally. Unicode is used in many technologies and operating systems. Unicode is promoted and supported by the Unicode Consortium. Unicode also allows private codes so users can assign values as needed.

Data Representation

Run Chart

The **run chart** is a line graph with a horizontal x axis (independent variables) and a vertical y axis (dependent variables, outcomes). The run chart, which provides a running record of a process over time, adds a horizontal median line, calculated according to the number of data points (data points + 1 divided by 2). A run is a sequence of data points on one side of the median line, ending when the line crosses the median. Runs may be color-coded. For example, a run chart may plot the number of urinary infections by month for a 1-year period with increased runs indicated by a different color. It is important that data be recorded for a long enough period that normal variations are not misconstrued as significant runs. Run charts (with more than twenty-five data points) may demonstrate shifts (eight points or more on one side of median line), trends (six data points in the same direction), and patterns (eight or more similar fluctuations). These changes point to specific causes that require investigation.

Control Chart

The **control chart** is similar to the run chart, but it has a mean line (the average of the data points) as well as upper and lower control limit lines, based on normal distribution. With any process, there is some normal variation (common cause or random variation) so the line values may vary; however, when the line crosses the control limits, this suggests that there is a specific cause (special cause variation) that requires investigation. The control limits are usually set at 2–3 standard deviations from the mean. Thus, the line shows the normal variations and excessive variations. The control chart can include horizontal lines, indicating each standard deviation for more precise information, dividing the graph into zones. Zone C is 1 standard deviation from the mean; zone B is 2 standard deviations from the mean; and zone A is 3 standard deviations from the mean. Positive values are above the mean line, and negative values are below. The data can be analyzed for specific trending, depending on the number of data points in each zone.

Trending Analysis

A **trending analysis** is applied to the run chart or control chart. In some cases, the data points on the chart may clearly go upward or downward, indicating a trend, but in other cases, there may be many variations, making the trend difficult to analyze. There are a number of rules applied to trending to help determine if variations are common-cause variations or special-cause variations:

- **Run (shift):** Seven or more consecutive data points are all above or all below the median (run chart) or mean (control chart).
- **Trend:** Seven or more consecutive data points are in either ascending or descending order with twenty-one or more total data points or six or more consecutive data points with fewer than twenty-one total data points.
- **Cycle:** An up and down variation forms a sawtooth pattern with fourteen successive data points, suggestive of a systemic effect on data. If the trend is related to common-cause variation, the variation may be demonstrated with four to eleven successive data points.
- **Astronomical value:** Data points unrelated to other points indicate a sentinel event or special-cause variation.

Balanced Scorecard

The **balanced scorecard** (designed by R. S. Kaplan and D. P. Norton) provides performance measures in relation to the mission and vision statement and goals and objectives. A balanced scorecard includes not only the traditional financial information but also data about customers, internal processes, and education/learning. Each organization can select measures that help to determine if the organization is on track to meeting its goals. These measures may include the following:

- **Customers:** types of customers and customer satisfaction.
- **Finances/business operations:** funding and cost-benefit analysis.
- **Clinical outcomes:** complications, infection rates, inpatient and outpatient data, and compliance with regulatory standards.
- **Education/learning:** in-service training, continuing education, assessment of learning, use of new skills, and research.
- **Community:** ongoing needs.
- **Growth:** innovative programs.

If the scorecard is adequately balanced, it reflects both the needs and priorities of the organization itself and also those of the community and customers.

Charts and Graphs

Presenting data in the form of **charts** and **graphs** provides a visual representation of the data that is easy to comprehend. There are basically three types of graphs: line graphs, bar graphs, and pie charts.

- **Line graphs** have an *x* and *y* axis; they are used to show how an independent variable affects a dependent variable. A line graph can be used to show the number of infections that occur each week, month, or year.
- **Bar graphs** are used to compare the relationship between two or more groups. The graphs can show quantifiable data as bars that extend horizontally, vertically, or stacked. Bar graphs can be used to show comparison data of different populations or data from one time period to another.
- **Pie charts** are used to show the percentage of an item as compared to the whole. A pie chart can show, for example, the distribution of infection-control resources.

Scattergram

A **scattergram** is a graphic display of the relationship between two variables with one variable plotted on the *x* axis and the other on the *y* axis. For example, the *x* axis may indicate age, and the *y* axis, admission to the emergency department. A data point is then entered for each admission, correlating with age. Analysis of the scattergram would then indicate the most common age distributions of patients. The scattergram can be used to test for possible cause–effect relationships, although this type of relationship is not required, and the scattergram is not proof of a correlation between data. As the data are plotted, repeat values are circled. With enough input, the data may begin to form a pattern. If this pattern is a straight line, there is evidence that there is a correlation between the two variables.

Dashboard

A **dashboard** (also called a digital dashboard), like the dashboard in a car, is an easy-to-read computer program that integrates a variety of performance measures or key indicators into one display (usually with graphs or charts) to provide an overview of an organization. It can include data regarding patient satisfaction, infection rates, financial status, or any other measurement that is important to assess performance. The dashboard provides a running picture of the status of a department or organization at any point in time and may be updated as needed—daily, weekly, or monthly. An organization-wide dashboard provides numerous benefits:

- Broad involvement of all departments
- A consistent and easy to understand visual representation of data
- Identification of negative findings or trends so that they can be corrected
- Availability of detailed reports
- Effective measurements that demonstrate the degree of efficiency

Assistance with making informed decisions

Display of Patient Data for Clinical Decision-Making

The effective **display of patient data** for clinical decision-making requires that information be rapidly available with minimal cognitive effort. The decision tree is a common presentation with potential options, consequences, and expected outcomes. Other types of presentations include tables, various types of graphs, and icons. In most cases, multiple modes of data presentation provide the best information. For example, if a health care provider wants to know a patient's trend in blood sugars, a line graph is effective; however, if the provider wants the exact numbers to determine insulin dosage, getting this information is easier from a table. Patient data should be integrated in a meaningful manner. For example, a change in heparin dosage should automatically display the latest prothrombin time/international normalized ratio for the patient. Visual indicators, such as different colors, may be used to highlight information, such as abnormal laboratory results. Pictorial displays can be effective, but multiple displays on one screen are distracting and slow the cognitive processing of data.

Patient Safety, Quality and Risk Management

Benchmarking

Benchmarking is an ongoing process of measuring practice, service, or product results against competitors or industry standards. The **Xerox Corporation** developed the **10-step benchmarking model**. This model compares an organization's efficiency with that of others and searches for improvements. The 10-step process moves through four phases: planning, analysis, integration, and action. The steps include the following:
- Identify benchmark targets.
- Identify organizations/units/providers with which to compare data.
- Determine and initiate methods of data collection.
- Evaluate current performance level and deficits.
- Project vision of future performance.
- Communicate findings and reach group agreement.
- Recommend changes based on benchmark data.
- Develop specific action plans for objectives.
- Implement actions and adjust as necessary based on monitoring of process.
- Update benchmarks based on latest data.

This basic benchmarking model is often modified to a 7–11-step process, depending on the needs of the organization. Benchmarking is often used to improve cash flow as health care becomes more competitive or to compare infection rates.

External Benchmarking and Internal Trending

External benchmarking involves analyzing data from outside an institution, such as monitoring national rates of hospital-acquired infection, and comparing them to internal rates. In order for this data to be meaningful, the same definitions must be used as well as the same populations or effective risk stratification. Using national data can be informative, but each institution is different; thus, relying on external benchmarking to select indicators for infection control, for example, can be misleading. Additionally, benchmarking is a compilation of data that may vary considerably if analyzed individually; it can be further compromised by anonymity, making comparisons difficult.

Internal trending involves comparing internal rates of one area or population with another, such as infection rates in intensive care units and general surgery; while this can help to pinpoint areas of concern within an institution, making comparisons is still problematic because of inherent differences. Using a combination of external and internal data can help to identify indicators.

Documentation of Quality Indicators

The Agency for Healthcare Research and Quality (AHRQ) provides software (current version 4.4) that allows tracking and **documentation of quality indicators (QIs)**; this software and focus on QIs can be integrated into the information system so that data can be easily accessed. The QI software programs of AHRQ include:
- SAS, which uses SAS/STAT statistical software (which is commercially available).
- Windows, which has a GUI and uses a SQL Server (which has a free version).

MONAHRQ, which facilitates development of a website for health care reporting, including data regarding quality of care, use, preventable hospitalizations, and rates for different conditions and procedures (free to federal, state, and local organizations). MONAHRQ is especially valuable for documenting QIs and providing access to consumers and health care providers because it is easy to use by downloading, inputting the organization's data, selecting options related to websites, and creating a website.

Terms Associated with Maintaining Quality Programs in Nursing

Programs to assess and maintain quality measures in nursing and many other areas revolve around a number of concepts. One is QA, or quality assurance, which a method to evaluate the degree of excellence by monitoring, evaluating and correcting problems if detected. Another term, less used perhaps in health care than in other fields, is total quality management, or TQM, which involves the formulation of an organizational mission statement encompassing the goal of satisfying the client. Total quality improvement (TQI) and continuous quality improvement (CQI) are concepts involving a continuous process of improvement. Nursing (and healthcare) tends to focus more on the last concept, which is performance improvement (PI). PI is a leadership-driven, organizational-focused process. For healthcare professionals, this typically means developing a process to design, measure, assess, and improve performance that can have a positive effect on patients.

Integration of Key Quality Concepts Within the Organization

There are a number of **key concepts** related to quality that must be communicated to all members of an organization through inservice, workshops, newsletters, fact sheets, and team meetings. Quality care/performance should be:
- **Appropriate** to needs and in keeping with best practices.
- **Accessible** to the individual despite financial, cultural, or other barriers.
- **Competent**, with practitioners well-trained and adhering to standards.
- **Coordinated** among all healthcare providers.
- **Effective** in achieving outcomes based on the current state of knowledge.
- **Efficient** in methods of achieving the desired outcomes.
- **Preventive**, allowing for early detection and prevention of problems.
- **Respectful** and caring with consideration of the individual needs given primary importance.
- **Safe** so that the organization is free of hazards or dangers that may put patients or others at risk.

Leapfrog Initiatives

Leapfrog is a consortium of health care purchasers/employers providing benefits to millions of Americans. The focus initially was on reducing health care costs by **preventing medical errors** and "leaping forward" by rewarding hospitals and health care organizations that improve safety and quality of care. Leapfrog has developed a number of **initiatives** to improve safety. These initiatives can be valuable tools in assessing and developing a patient safety culture. Leapfrog provides an annual Hospital and Quality Safety Survey to assess progress, releases regional data, and encourages voluntary public reporting. Leapfrog has instituted the Leapfrog Hospital Rewards Program as a pay-for-performance program to reward organizations for showing improvement in key measures. One initiative includes preventing medical errors. Purchasers of health care agree to the base purchase of health care based on four principals:

- Educating enrollees about patient safety and providing comparative performance data
- Recognizing and rewarding health care organizations that demonstrate improvement in preventing errors
- Making health plans accountable for implementing these principles
- Advocating for these principles with clients by using benefits consultants

Leapfrog has developed a number of specific **initiatives** related to **safe practices**, including:

- Implementation of a computerized physicians order entry system that includes software to detect and prevent errors with a goal of decreasing prescribing errors by more than 50%.
- Evidence-based hospital referral, requiring referral to hospitals that demonstrate the best results with high-risk conditions and surgeries; these are assessed, according to the number of procedures or treatments done each year and outcome data with a goal of reducing mortality rates by 40%.
- Intensive care unit physician staffing requiring specially trained specialists (intensivists) with a goal of reducing mortality rates by 40%.

Leapfrog Safe Practices Score, which assesses the progress a health care organization makes on thirty safe practices that Leapfrog has identified as reducing the risk of harm to patients.

Institute of Medicine and National Committee for Quality Assurance Safety Issues

The **Institute of Medicine (IOM)**, founded in 1970 under the charter of the National Academy of Sciences, is a nonprofit organization that serves an advisory role on health care issues to governmental and nongovernmental decision-makers. The IOM advises the government but is outside of the governmental structure to ensure lack of bias. The IOM issues guidelines based on research and evidence, conducts studies for Congress and other organizations, and conducts a number of epidemiological studies. The IOM is involved in a broad range of activities, issues regular reports, and provides workshops and forums about a health care issues (e.g., obesity). The IOM has standing committees to focus on specific issues and provide forums for general discussion. Additionally, the IOM provides fellowships to help professionals gain experience and expertise in health-related fields.

The **Institute of Medicine** called for accrediting agencies to ensure organizations focus on patient safety. In response, the **National Committee for Quality Assurance** has addressed safety issues as part of its accreditation standards. Guidelines directed at managed care organizations provide useful information for other organizations as well. Organizations should:

- Educate staff regarding clinical safety by providing information.
- Provide collaborative training within the network related to safe clinical practice.
- Combine data within the network (organization) on adverse outcomes and polypharmacy.
- Make improving patient safety a priority for quality improvement activities.

Provide and distribute information about safe practices that includes information about computerized pharmacy order systems, physicians trained in intensive care, best practices, and research on safe clinical practices.

Agency for Healthcare Research and Quality and Evidence-Based Practice Centers

The **Agency for Healthcare Research and Quality** promotes evidence-based practice through funding of **evidence-based practice centers (EPCs)** to develop evidence-based practice guidelines for dissemination and use in development of patient care plans, establishing insurance coverage, and development of educational materials. These centers issue research reports, including meta-analysis of all relevant research, on a wide range of topics, such as "Pain Management Interventions for Elderly Patients with Hip Fracture," which include morbidity/mortality rates and cost-effectiveness associated with different treatments and procedures. Research focuses on areas of significance to people receiving Medicaid and Medicare. For example, five EPCs are engaging in research on technology for the Centers for Medicaid and Medicare, which focuses on topics related to the U.S. Preventive Services Task Force. Partners, such as insurance companies, professional associations, patient advocacy groups, and employers, nominate topics. Guides are available for both consumers and clinicians.

The **quality indicators (QIs)** from the **Agency for Healthcare Research and Quality** are distributed as a software tool free of charge to health care organizations to help them identify adverse events or potential adverse events that require further study. This software is an invaluable aid in assessing and developing the organization's patient safety culture. Current quality indicators include the following:

- **Prevention QIs** use patient discharge data to determine conditions that require ambulatory care to prevent rehospitalization.
- **Inpatient QIs** measure quality of care through types of procedures, use of procedures, and mortality rates associated with procedures or conditions.
- **Patient Safety QIs** use data regarding adverse events and complications related to surgeries, medical procedures, and childbirth.
- **Pediatric QIs** use patient discharge data to screen for problems related to pediatric exposure to health care and analyze system changes that may prevent problems.

The data indicators may also be used to assess safety factors at an area (e.g., county) level per 100,000 population.

National Quality Forum

The **National Qualify Forum (NQF)** has endorsed a set of safe practices that can be used to assess and develop the organization's patient safety culture. Practices encompass creating a safe culture as well as specific steps to ensure safe practices throughout the organization. According to NQF, the four elements needed to create and sustain a patient safety culture include the following:
- Leadership must ensure structures are in place for organization-wide awareness and compliance with safety measures, including adequate resources and direct accountability.
- Measurement, analysis, and feedback must track safety and allow for interventions.
- Team-based patient care with adequate training and performance improvement activities must be organization-wide.
- Safety risk must be continuously identified and interventions taken to reduce patient risk.

National Quality Forum's safe practices include:
- Considering patient's rights/responsibilities, providing informed consent, respecting advance directives, making full disclosure of medical errors, managing information and care by documenting care properly, providing prompt accurate test results, using standard procedures for labeling diagnostic studies, & providing discharge planning.
- Managing medications by implementing a computerized prescriber order entry system, standardizing abbreviations, maintaining updated medication lists for patients/pharmacists in medication management, identifying high-alert drugs, and dispensing drugs in unit doses.
- Providing adequate well-trained and well-supervised staff and resources, including critical care physicians.
- To prevent HCA infections: ventilate properly, central lines, wash hands, immunize, & surgical care procedures.
- Providing safe practices for surgery, i.e., informing patient of risks, taking measures to prevent errors, and using prophylactic treatments to prevent complications.
- Providing procedures/ongoing assessment to prevent adverse events, such as pressure ulcers, thromboembolism/DVT, allergic reactions, or anticoagulation complications.

Close-Call Events

Close-call events are those events that could have led to an error or patient injury but were detected in time to prevent the error/injury. For example, if a nurse delivers the wrong dose of medication to a patient but notices the error before administration, this is a close-call event. Close-call events caused by informatics can occur if patients' names are not clearly displayed resulting in access of the wrong patient record. Key information that is not easily accessible or prominently displayed may result in errors. Incorrect dosages may be assigned if the dosage is not easily readable. Errors are likely to increase with poor EHR design, system downtime, inadequate training, and incomplete implementation. Free-text instructions (such as to hold a medication) that are not programmed into the CPOE may lead to overdosage. Informatics may help prevent error through user-friendly design, check and balance systems (including virus detection programs, backup paper forms, offsite backup, and redundant systems), alarms, and alerts.

Failure Mode and Effects Analysis

Failure mode and effects analysis (FMEA) is a team-based prospective analysis method that attempts to identify and correct failures in a process before utilization to ensure positive outcomes and is especially valuable to detect the potential for errors in electronic health records and other health information technology. Steps include:
- Definition: Process description.
- Team creation.
- Description: Flow charts showing each step and sub-step in process.
- Brainstorming: Each step and sub-step brainstormed for potential failure modes.
- Identification and recording of potential causes of potential failures: Utilizing cause and effect diagram, root cause analysis.
- Listing potential adverse outcomes.
- Assignment of severity rating: Potential adverse outcomes rated (1-10 scale, slight to death).
- Assignment of frequency/occurrence rating: Potential failures rated on 1-10 scale with (1 remote = 1:10,000 and 10 very high) within a specified time period, usually a year.
- Assignment of detection rating (scale of 1-10): Potential failures rated (1-10 scale) on likelihood hazards, errors, or failures will be identified prior to occurrence.
- Calculation of risk priority number: Based on scales of severity, occurrence, and detection.
- Reduction of potential failures.
- Identification of performance measures.

Hardware Device Selection

Hospital Information Systems (HIS)

Information systems dedicated to medical facilities are known as **Hospital Information Systems (HIS)**. Typically, HIS use a mainframe computer (server) with satellite terminals (or workstations) located throughout the facility. These terminals may be hardwired together (or linked using a local area network (LAN)) to communicate with the central server. There are three broad types of HIS: administrative, semi-clinical, and clinical:

- **Administrative:** handle non-medical management issues such as payroll.
- **Semi-clinical:** partly administrative and partly medical.
  - Tracks the flow of patients into and out of the hospital.
  - Performs order-entry results reporting.
- **Clinical:** handles medical issues.
  - Point-of-Service (POS): information is entered directly into the system at the patient's bedside rather than having the information transcribed from written notes.
  - Specialty Support Programs: there are many systems currently available that support healthcare facility issues such as laboratory, pharmacy, and radiology.

Computer Hardware and Peripherals

Computer Hardware: Computers are used to make complex calculations, store information, and speed data processing. Within the medical field, computers were first used only in the areas of billing, payroll, and scheduling. They are now used in nearly every aspect of medical care. Computers contain physical parts known as hardware. Hardware is usually housed inside a plastic case, but there may be components that exist outside of the case. The computer case usually houses the motherboard, microchips, processors, and electronic circuits that carry out the computer's primary functions.

The following are the **major internal types of hardware** of all computers:

- The **motherboard** is a thin piece of non-conducting plastic onto which the computer's circuits are printed. The motherboard also has areas where chips are mounted and slots are placed which allow the addition of other pieces of hardware.
- The **central processing unit (CPU)** is comprised of different unit types: arithmetic, logic, control, and memory. Arithmetic and logic units control the computer's mathematical functions and test Boolean logic.
- **Control units** perform fetch, execute, decode, and store functions based on the computer's machine language. Fetch is the process of retrieving information from storage. Decode is the process of making that information useable. Execute is the process of sending the decoded information to the arithmetic and logic unit. Store is the process of putting the resulting information into the computer's memory.

Peripherals: This term encompasses the hardware that is connected to the computer to make it fully functional. Peripherals include the keyboard, printer, monitor, storage devices, and mouse. Storage devices include disk drives, hard drives, and USB drives.

Some commonly used peripherals include:

- **Light pen:** A light pen can highlight information and send data to the computer by touching a specially designed monitor that recognizes the pen.
- **Touch screens:** Touch screens allow the user to physically tap the screen with their finger or a plastic pen device in order to make choices.
- **Optical character recognition (OCR):** OCR allows data to be read by a special device directly from the source. This technology is used in grocery store checkouts and standardized test grading. A similar form of input reader is the magnetic-ink character recognition (MICR). Banks use MICR to read the routing and account numbers of checks.
- **Computer enhanced imaging:** Computer enhanced imaging is of particular importance to the medical field. Two examples include CAT scans (computerized axial tomography) and MRI (magnetic resonance imaging).

Input and Output Devices

Input devices: Information is delivered to a computer via input devices. Examples of common input devices include keyboard, mouse, scanner, touch screen, light pen, and even the human voice. Some less common examples of input devices include security scanners for fingerprints, retinal prints, voiceprints, electrodes, optical scanners; magnetic-ink character recognition readers; MRIs; and CAT scans.

Output devices: Information that is provided from the computer flows through output devices. Output devices send this information to where it can be seen or heard. The printer, monitor, and speakers are all output devices. Additionally, the computer can send various signals to receiving units to allow for status checks, abnormal conditions, or security breeches.

Some peripherals can be used for both input and output, including CD-ROM's, DVDs, and USB drives (sometimes referred to as thumb drives).

Bits and Bytes

Computers use binary code to store data. Binary code has only two conditions: zero (off) and one (on). This is because early computers used physical relay switches with an on or off switch. A **bit** (binary digit) is defined as a single symbol of the binary code (its value equals zero or one). These bits are arranged into an eight-symbol unit (called a **byte**) to code meaningful information such as letters of the alphabet or numbers. From a series of eight bits, 255 different combinations of bytes can be formed. The cost of computer memory has come down in recent years and most home computers come with a minimum of 512 mega-bytes (MB) of main (active) memory, and a hard drive that can store 60 gigabytes (GB) of data.

Major Classes of Computers

There are three major **classes** of computers:
- **Analog:** Analog computers measure specific continuous data and do not break the information down any further. They may measure temperature, pressure, heart rate, voltage, or current. The fetal monitor is one example of an analog computer used by nurses.
- **Digital:** Digital computers use binary code to represent data. This is the most common type of computer used at home and in businesses. Networked computers also communicate using binary code.
- **Hybrid:** Hybrid computers have elements of both analog and digital computers. These computers are produced and used for highly specific tasks which are often based on physics and engineering. The ECG and EEG are two types of hybrid computers. They take analog inputs (brain waves in the case of the EEG) and transcribe them into binary data so that they can be studied and compared using a digital computer.

Hardware Required for a Computer Network

Computers that are linked to a server or network must have a network adapter (or network interface card) and a data pathway to communicate with the server or network. The most common network interface card (NIC) is called an ethernet card. An ethernet card (or alternative network adapter) is installed onto a networked computer and allows full time access to the local area network (LAN). The data connection can be accomplished either through a wired connection, such as an attached ethernet cable, or a wireless connection, established with one or more network access points (wireless routers).

Hardware Limitations

Technical specifications or requirements are usually described in detail, including operational characteristics and **limitations**. Technical specifications may include operations, operating system, version, display requirements, software requirements, capacities, features, devices, connections, supported environments, and data sources. Understanding the limitations of hardware is necessary for installation and use. Limitations may relate to the equipment (e.g., an inability to do some functions, standards, nonpermitted devices, limited number of slave devices), requirements (e.g., operating system, software packages that must be installed, type of power supply, environmental temperature), system managers (e.g., support not provided if operating system or equipment is modified, types of reports that can and cannot be generated), and users (e.g., help function limited to specific criteria, limits in access, sequence of key strokes for specific actions).

System Software

There are two types of **software**: system and application. They are defined as follows:

- **System software:** System software includes the programs that instruct the computer how to run. Utility software may also be included under the definition of system software. The basic input/output system (BIOS) is encoded directly onto a computer chip and activates each time the computer is started. Basic input output system is sometimes referred to as firmware. The BIOS finds and loads the computer's operating system (OS) into the random access memory (RAM). The OS manages the storage of data on the central processing unit (CPU), the interaction between CPU and peripherals, and the interaction between user and computer. The original user-computer interface was DOS (disk operating system). Disk operating system was a programming language that was difficult to learn and made home computer use impractical. The first graphical user interface (GUI) came onto the market in 1984 and is the standard for all personal computers today.
- **Application software:** Application software is targeted to the end-user and allows the user to conduct computer-aided processes such as word processing or spreadsheets.

Utility Programs for Computers

Utility programs provide enhancements to the overall computing environment. Antivirus software (which protects against attacks from malicious code) is one type of utility program. Language translation software and web browsers are also classified as utility programs. Language translation utilities (also known as assembler, compilers, or interpreters) work to translate human language into binary code that can be understood by the computer. Web browsers (Chrome, Firefox, Edge, etc) create a graphical user interface (GUI) simplifying internet access and use.

Trends

Cloud Computing

Cloud computing is using the internet to store and access files as opposed to a business network or a computer hard drive. Cloud computing has dramatically increased by healthcare organizations in the past years, likely associate with health care reform giving financial incentives for providers and organizations that use electronic medical records and electronic health records (EHR). Health care organizations are also using the cloud to store information that is not EHR related at rapidly increasing numbers. The benefits to using the cloud include multiple providers being able to access the records at the same time from many different locations, increasing collaboration and decreasing healthcare costs. The major disadvantages focus on privacy concerns, as patient's personal health information is being stored on the internet, making it susceptible to cybercriminals. As the health care industry moves to new and alternative solutions to satisfy the "meaningful use" clause given by the Centers for Medicare and Medicaid Services, cloud providers are coming up with new agreements to protect private information, thereby becoming more attractive to healthcare organizations.

Advantages and Disadvantages of Using the Internet as Part of an Organization's Information System

The following is a list of **advantages** of using the **internet** as part of an organization's information system:
- End users only need a basic computer with internet connectivity to use the information system.
- Web browser software is readily available and free.
- Maintenance and upgrades occur at a central location, elevating the need to upgrade everyone's individual computer.
- Internet access is broadly available, faster, and more dependable.
- The connection can also be used for webcasts, email, and voice communications.
- Access to the internet allows users to conduct independent research and troubleshoot problems.

The following is a list of **disadvantages** of using the **internet** as part of an organization's information system:
- Connectivity quality is different from one site to another (e.g., connection speed, browser compatibility, etc.).
- A web portal must be developed that has security features such as a firewall and high-level encryption capabilities.
- A web portal is open 24 hours a day, 7 days a week to potential hackers and unscrupulous personnel.
- The information system is vulnerable to technical issues that occur at the supplier of the internet connections (ISP).
- Employees may use the internet connection for purposes other than work.

mHealth

As computers become more prevalent, smaller, and more powerful, they can be used in more facets of everyday life. This advance of technology has allowed for a new sector in healthcare known as

mHealth. Mobile computers and wireless communication technology work together to improve the way healthcare is delivered. This trend has grown as mobile systems have become less expensive and wireless communication becomes more widespread. Devices used in mHealth include diabetes monitors, IV delivery systems, and fetal dopplers. These intelligent devices are networked into mHealth systems. The way these devices communicate is to use standard computer communication standards. The standards that are at the forefront of this technology include digitized voice, third-generation broadband, and packet-based transmission. This technology allows patients to have real time control and monitoring of their medical conditions.

Wireless Technology

Most modern computer information systems operate at least partially on **wireless technology**. Wireless computing, in the form of wireless local area networks (Wi-Fi) and devices such as smartphones and tablets enable healthcare workers to send and receive information at the same place where they care for the patient. The major benefits to doing this include:
- There is less chance of human error.
- There is less chance of information being seen by unauthorized personnel.
- There is a savings in time.
- Human error is decreased because the necessity of having to transcribe information into a patient's chart from the physician written or spoken notes is eliminated.
- Computer files are generally more secure than paper charts because they are accessed only with a user identification number and password so only authorized personnel can gain access to them.
- Since information is directly input into the system, files are updated immediately, which eliminates the significant amount of time that was previously needed to manually update files.

Wearable Devices

Use of healthcare-related **wearable devices** has increased markedly in the past few years and will continue to do so because large companies, such as Samsung, is focusing on producing products for the healthcare industry. Patients are especially likely to use devices recommended by healthcare professionals. Devices include:
- **Smart Glove, smart boards, and game-based technology:** Used to measure motion and help to create exercises specific to patients with neurological or musculoskeletal injuries.
- **Glucose monitoring devices:** Watch-like devices use microneedles to assess and display blood glucose levels.
- **Temperature monitoring devices:** Available in a variety of different types of devices. May provide remote monitoring through smartphones.
- **Pain monitors:** Measure EEG changes and provide distracting content, such as music or videos, or medication.
- **Cardiac monitoring systems:** Transmit data through smartphone or other devices.
- **Virtual reality**: Used to train staff and to promote relaxation and mobility in patients.
- **Fertility monitors:** Watch-like device tracks fertility and menstrual cycle when worn during the night.

Integrating Social Media Elements to Benefit Patients

Applying **social media elements** to healthcare technology allows patient interaction. This can provide valuable information to healthcare providers so that they can better care for patients and may increase patients' participation and satisfaction. Social media elements include:

- **Sharing data:** Patients may access a patient portal to view laboratory reports and other records.
- **Messaging/Emailing:** Reminders and alerts can be sent to patients regarding appointments or guidelines. May be used inhouse to reduce the number of audible pages in order to provide a quieter environment.
- **Surveying:** Surveys can be sent to patients immediately after treatment or discharge in order to assess their status and their satisfaction with care.
- **Transmitting photographs:** Patients can submit photographs to healthcare providers, such as a picture of a rash, to assist with telephone triage or assessment.
- **Using Facebook/Twitter:** Information about the healthcare provider may be provided in order to reach a large population. Facebook may allow comments, but these should be monitored before publication.

Telehealth

Telehealth refers to the delivery of healthcare services to patients who are not physically present with the healthcare professional, usually due to remote location or disability. Telehealth can be delivered over a telephone, via e-mail, or by video conference. The primary benefits of telehealth are that it allows for the extension of precious healthcare resources, lowers the overall cost of healthcare, and allows patients to receive healthcare who would not normally have access to it. There are a number of ways in which telehealth is useful to healthcare professionals:

- Consultation with colleagues.
- Patient interviews.
- Monitor a patient's biometric values and assess their condition.
- Evaluate diagnostic images, which allows physicians to remotely view and evaluate these images even if they are located overseas (e.g., India).
- Evaluation of microscope slides and laboratory reports.

One of the most valuable trends in medicine today is **telehealth**. Compared to telemedicine, telehealth includes prevention and promotion of healthier lifestyles in addition to the curative focus of telemedicine. Thanks to the prevalence of personal computers and internet access, doctors can consult with one another, share information in real-time, or make "virtual house calls" in which they are able to both speak to and view the patient over an internet connection. Virtual house calls can help patients with many illnesses. For example, clients with diabetes can be coached to manage their diet and exercise regime at home.

One way that doctors can consult is through the use of intraoperative monitoring (IOM) during surgery. Intraoperative monitoring allows a specially trained surgeon to constantly monitor a patient remotely during the operation. Using IOM, surgery can be performed in one location while the IOM specialist monitors the patient from afar. This reduces the risk of patient death or complications.

There are many patient benefits associated with the use of **telehealth**. Several are outlined below:
- The patient does not have to travel to seek the advice of specialists who may be located many miles away.
- Electronic healthcare records can be accessed anywhere and at anytime. This access must be balanced with the privacy needs of individual patients and regulations (e.g., HIPAA).
- The patient becomes an active member in his or her own health care.
- Healthcare professionals from many different disciplines are able to collaborate and decide on the most appropriate course of action for the patient.
- Patients and family members have access to educational materials that are useful in helping the patient manage their condition.
- More patients have access to a specialist.
- Reduces or eliminates the cost of travel and thereby lowers the overall cost of healthcare.
- Digital records are easily accessible by healthcare providers.

Grand Rounds

Grand rounds have traditionally been a primary teaching tool for healthcare professionals. In grand rounds, a group of healthcare practitioners looks over a patient's case history and current condition. They then work together to develop a treatment plan.

Using **telehealth** (faxes, e-mails, and video conferencing), individuals scattered from one another can work together for the benefit of both students and patients involved with grand rounds. Two major benefits of using this process are: (1) lower costs due to the participants not having to travel to a specific location: (2) allow a wider audience of healthcare trainees, experts, and patients to participate in grand rounds.

This is an example of how technology can leverage resources to benefit patients. As healthcare resources become more rationed due to budgetary constraints, tools such as telehealth become more important.

Online Resources for Healthcare Needs

The following **online resources** are an extension of modern telehealth:
- Access to published guidelines of current standards of care. This includes news and discussions by medical experts.
- Critical pathways for help in deciding a patient's course of care. A patient can research their condition and receive information from many different sources.
- Information on drugs including: cost, effectiveness, and side effects. Patients can also research generic equivalent drugs (or drug combinations) that can help with the high cost of brand name prescription drugs.
- Electronic prescriptions, which lower the incidence of fraud and help with insurance claims. This also allows the prescription to be delivered to the patient's door.
- Patients may also search for journal articles and relevant medical literature related to their condition.
- Bulletin boards and discussion groups are active on many healthcare related subjects.

IDEATel, RLI, and Health Buddy

Three specific applications of telehealth currently in use are:
- **IDEATel,** the Diabetes Education and Telemedicine Project, was started in February 2000. This program uses aggressive monitoring to track patients' blood glucose values and enables physicians to make small changes in the medication plan on a day-to-day basis.
- **RLI**, Resource Link of Iowa, works with the chronically ill in Iowa. Patients are given a two-way interactive video device that allows them to have a high level of care while lowering the number of in person appointments with healthcare workers.
- **Health Buddy** is a small electronic appliance that asks the patient questions, sends reminders, and communicates medical information to the physician. Several other devices, such as a glucose monitor, can be directly linked to the Health Buddy for ease in transferring data.

Using Telehealth for Home-Based Healthcare

There are a number of ways that **telehealth** can be used for **home healthcare:**
- A home health nurse can transmit important information (such as wound photos) to a specialized nurse instead of requiring the specialist to visit the patient in the home. This type of practice reduces costs and allows more patients to be cared for appropriately.
- Family members who are struggling with caring for their ill loved ones can use the internet to find information and support, easing their fears and lowering their stress levels.
- Round the clock monitoring of diabetics, post-operative patients, and women with high-risk pregnancies can be achieved while the patients remain in the comfort of their own home thanks to the technology that allows biometric measurements to be sent directly to their healthcare facility.
- Geriatric patients can have regular videoconferences with any number of healthcare professionals allowing them to remain in their own home instead of moving into a long-term facility.

Telenursing

A subset of telehealth, **telenursing** is defined by the National Council of State Boards of Nursing (NCSBN) as "the practice of nursing over distance using telecommunication technology." In this case, telecommunications includes telephone, fax, and the internet.

Although this type of nursing has been in practice for decades, it was not until the mid 1990s that the NCSBN formulated its definition and set practical rules of liability regarding its practice. The NCSBN recognized that a nurse does not have to physically be present with a patient to practice nursing. It found that telenursing forms the legal status of "duty to care" and must be regulated. One problem with regulating telenursing involves the complexity that the patient may be in one state and the nurse in another. This may cause regulatory violations due to individual state's laws. This example shows the importance of creating uniform nationwide regulation of telehealth in general.

Clinical Devices

Electronic Beds

Electronic beds include:
- **Circo-electric beds:** Beds that rotate so that patients who cannot be moved can be placed in different positions to relieve pressure, facilitate interactions, and promote circulation.
- **Low air loss beds:** Allow air that is pumped in the support surface to leak, so there is a continuous flow of air through the air pillows in the device. The air pressure in the pillows in the devices can be adjusted according to the individual needs.
- **Air-fluidized (high air loss) beds:** Special bed systems that have a high flow of air through silicon beads, originally designed for treatment of burn patients. As the air flows through the beads, it "fluidizes" them so that they move, and provide support and redistribution of pressure in much the way water does. The beads are contained in a bathtub-like frame. The lower part of the body becomes immersed in the beads.
- **Smart beds:** May include motion alarms and motion-activated night lights and may provide verbal warnings, such as "Please, do not get out of bed" and "Your call light is not connected."

Intravenous Infusion Pumps and Smart Pumps

Intravenous infusion pumps allow IV fluids and medications to be delivered in a preset volume and at a preset rate. Alarms will sound if the infusion changes speed, stops, or finishes but if the settings were programmed incorrectly, the infusion pump does not correct this. Smart pumps, however, provide additional safety.

Smart pumps include infusion pumps for large volumes and syringes as well as for patient-controlled analgesia. Smart pumps are programmable and sound alarms if problems, such as completion of an IV, arise. Smart pumps are increasingly sophisticated and some can interact with the patient's electronic health record as well as the CPOE and barcode medication scanner. Some have built-in drug libraries (error reduction software) to monitor dosage and frequency of drugs. Smart pumps reduce errors, but they can still be programmed incorrectly and alarms ignored or overridden, so they are not error proof.

Barcode Medication Administration

Barcode medication administration (BCMA) uses wireless mobile units at the point of care to scan the barcode on each unit of medication or blood component before it is dispensed. Scanning ensures the correct medication and dosage is given to the correct patient, eliminating most point of administration medication errors. The BCMA system can also be used for specimen collection. This system requires monitoring and input from the pharmacy, as each new barcode must be entered into the system. Additionally, some medications are received in bulk, so when they are dispensed in unit doses, barcodes must be individually attached. Staff must be trained to ensure that BCMA is used properly and consistently. The Food and Drug Administration has required that drug supplies provide barcodes on the labels of medications and other biological product. BCMA increases safety for patients, integrates with the medication administration record, and the information system of the organization, providing data for assessment.

Biomedical Device Interfaces

Biomedical devices, such as physiological monitors (heart rate, blood pressure) and smart pumps, must **interface** between the patient and the device and then in digital form from the device to the information system, which must aggregate the data, which are then sent to an interface that converts the data to HL7 for transmission to the electronic health record. While standardization is occurring, there are at present many communication standards, and interfacing with older systems or modified systems poses problems. Additionally, interface requirements vary among devices. Elements that must be considered in determining interoperability of biomedical devices include the following:

- Type of device, including manufacturer and specifications.
- Network connectivity capabilities and whether the device is part of the same or a different network.
- Wired (specifications) or wireless (Bluetooth, 802.11, others).
- Transport, data, messaging, and certifications (Continua, ICE).
- Type of data transmitted by the device.
- Extra equipment required, such as a dongle, for connection or cables.
- Security of data.

Sleep Monitors, Smart Watches, Smart Heart Monitors, and Fitness Trackers

Medical smart devices include:

- **Sleep/Vital statistics monitors:** A disk is placed under the patient's mattress to detect sleeping patterns, heartrate, respiratory rate, and movements.
- **Smart watches:** These devices connect to smart phones, and applications may be used to detect seizures; monitor daily activity and exercise; monitor cardiac status, heart rate and rhythm; monitor tremors; monitor diabetes status and need for insulin; monitor medications (including alarms to note time to take medications); monitor eating behaviors; and monitor emotional status.
- **Smart heart monitors**: Some, such as Duo®, include a digital stethoscope and portable ECG to continuously monitor a patient's cardiac status. A coded chest strap is included, and the monitor is available in a watch-like device. Another commonly used device is the Zio XT patch, which provides up to 2 weeks of continuous ECG data. The device is small and adheres to the chest wall so it can be used during any type of activity, including showers.
- **Fitness trackers:** Watch-like device allows users to track activities, such as the number of daily steps, and some include heartrate monitoring. Data may or may not be transmitted to a smartphone or computer, depending on cost and complexity.

Clinical Decision Support Systems

Clinical decision support systems (CDSSs) are intended for the end user and comprise interactive software applications that provide information to physicians or other health care providers to help with health care decisions. The programs contain a base of medical knowledge to which patient data can be entered so an evidence-based inference system can provide patient-specific advice. For example, a CDSS system may be used in the Emergency Department so that staff can enter symptoms into the program and, based on the information entered, the CDSS program provides possible diagnoses and treatment options.

The CDSS system may be used for a variety of purposes, such as:
- Record keeping and documentation, such as authorization.
- Monitoring of patient's treatments, research protocols, orders, and referrals.
- Ensuring cost-effectiveness by monitoring orders to prevent duplication or tests that are not indicated by the condition or by presenting symptoms.
- Providing support in physician diagnosis and ensuring treatment is based on best practices.

Alerts Component of Clinical Decision Support Systems

Clinical decision support (CDS) systems may include general information as well as guidelines regarding treatment and medications based on symptoms or diagnosis. **Alerts** are an important component of CDSs and may be used for cost-effectiveness, safety, and preventive health. Alerts should not be excessive, which results in "fatigue" with users ignoring or overriding repeated alerts.

Types of alerts may include the following:
- Warnings regarding medication interactions
- Reminders for preventive actions, such as routine scheduling of mammogram
- Notification of duplicate testing
- Activation of help wizard to assist the user

Issues to consider with alerts include whether or not:
- The data are accurate enough to avoid inappropriate alerts.
- The data can be overridden (e.g., ignoring a drug–drug interaction) and what types of alerts can be overridden.
- An alert should apply to all patients or to a select group, such as those with a particular diagnosis.
- Alerts focus on reminding users to use an order or warning them to avoid an order.
- Viewing the alert requires activation or is automatic.

Computerized Provider Order Entry Systems

Computerized provider order entry (CPOE) systems greatly reduce paperwork and decrease errors. The system allows healthcare providers to enter prescription information or treatment orders via the computer. Once the information has been entered directly into the computer, it is checked for a wide variety of potential errors including: drug interactions, drug allergies, and patient condition alerts. The benefits of CPOE include:
- **Patient centered**: Changes are made in real-time and make for the safest treatment possible.
- **Intuitive**: The interface resembles a paper document and can be personalized for an individual provider.
- **Secure**: Meets all regulatory guidelines for secure access thanks to the use of electronic signatures.
- **Portable**: No matter where a patient is seen throughout the United Sates, their healthcare provider can access their information.
- Computerized provider order entry systems make **billing easier and more accurate** since the system codes the diagnosis at the time of entry.

Computerized Physician Order Entry

Computerized physician order entry (CPOE) is a clinical software application that automates medication/treatment ordering, requiring that orders be typed in a standard format to avoid mistakes in ordering or interpreting orders. CPOE is promoted by Leapfrog as a means to reduce medication errors. About 50% of medication errors occur during ordering, so reducing this number can have a large impact on patient safety. Most CPOE systems contain a clinical decision support system as well so that the system can provide an immediate alert related to patient allergies, drug interactions, duplicate orders, or incorrect dosing at the time of data entry. Some systems can also provide suggestions for alternative medications, treatments, and diagnostic procedures. The CPOE system may be integrated into the information system of the organization for easier tracking of information and data collection. This system is cost-effective, replaces handwritten orders, and allows easy access to patient records.

Types of Computer Networks

There are four types of computer **networks**:
- **Local area networks:** Local area networks (LANs) are often used by companies to connect the computers in a single area or building. Local area networks are typically connected to a server (or servers) located in the same building.
- **Metropolitan area networks:** Metropolitan area networks (MANs) are used to connect computers on a university campus or local government agencies housed in separate buildings within the same general area. These networks are typically wired with ethernet.
- **Wide area networks:** Wide area networks (WANs) connect computers that are separated by a large geographical space such as individual hospitals owned by the same company. Wide area networks are typically connected via a virtual private network (VPN).
- **Internet:** The internet is a worldwide network of computers accessed by an internet service provider.

Architecture and Topology

The terms architecture and topology are defined as follows:
- **Architecture:** In the field of informatics, architecture is defined by the type of computer system used. Network architecture is the form of communication used between the computers involved. Broadcast communication, typically used in local area networks (LANs), involves sending the same data to every computer in the network. For example, a connection to the internet consists of point-to-point communication where one computer sends information to only the specified computer.
- **Topology:** The way that computers are interconnected in a LAN is known as topology. When computers are connected to the network by a direct line, this is called bus topology. Star topology relies on a central computer (called a server) to relay information to each separate computer. Early local area networks were built on a ring topology (all computers were directly connected with one another).

Voice-Over Internet Protocol

Voice-over Internet Protocol (VoIP) includes the protocols and technology involved in allowing audio and multimedia transmission, such as audio, FAX, messaging, and short-messaging service (SMS), which is text messaging, over the internet. VoIP is also referred to as broadband telephone or internet telephone, and companies, such as Vonage, market their service as an alternative to landline telephones. VoIP technology encodes audio into digital files for streaming transmission, using a number of codecs. VoIP allows SMS or calls from non-phone devices with access to Wi-Fi, 3G, or 4G. A number of network protocols are in use, but Session Description Protocol is common. Many organizations are switching to VoIP devices and eliminating landline telephones as a cost-saving measure because voice and data can use the same network.

Radio-Frequency Identification

Radio-frequency identification (RFID) is an automatic system for identification that employs embedded digital memory chips with unique codes to track patients, medical devices, medications, and staff. A chip can carry multiple types of data, such as expiration dates, patient's allergies, and blood types. A chip/tag may, for example, be embedded in the identification bracelet of the patient, and all medications for the patient are tagged with the same chip. Chips have the ability to both read and write data, so they are more flexible than bar coding. The data on the chips can be read by sensors from a distance or through materials, such as clothes, although tags do not apply or read well on metal or in fluids. There are two types of RFID:

- **Active:** Continuous signals are transmitted between the chips and sensors.
- **Passive:** Signals are transmitted when in proximity to a sensor.

Thus, a passive system may be adequate for administration of medications, but an active system would be needed to track movements of staff, equipment, or patients.

Bluetooth Technology

Bluetooth technology is proprietary technology developed by Ericsson and managed by Bluetooth Special Interest Group (SIG), which has established Bluetooth standards and oversees use. While this is considered open technology, licensing is required for permission to use various patents. Bluetooth is wireless technology that allows the use of short-wave radio transmissions (ISM 2400-2480 MHz) to exchange data in fixed devices and mobile devices, such as cell phones, faxes, global position system receivers, digital cameras, and computers. The user can create personal area networks that are secure. The master-slave concept is used with Bluetooth technology, so the "master" (primary device) can communicate with up to seven other "slave" devices, although the roles of master and slave are interchangeable. Range is usually relatively short but can vary. A typical example of a Bluetooth device is the hands-free headset. Bluetooth is intended primarily for portable devices.

Digital Picture Archiving and Communication Systems

Due to the logarithmic trend in affordable computer memory, memory intensive applications such as digital photos or video are now mainstream. **Picture archiving and communication systems (PACS)** have lead the way towards a "filmless" medical system. Digital images take the place of traditional radiological film. The system is able to acquire, display, send, and store digital images. Picture archiving and communication systems are used in a large number of radiology including mammography, magnetic resonance imaging, endoscopy, and X-rays. These systems allow practitioners to view and report on images without any restrictions on time and distance. It is important that PACS be integrated with any existing or planned information system in the organization. Picture archiving and communication systems save time and resources and are a very good investment for healthcare organizations.

Healthcare Data Encryption

Data encryption uses algorithms to scramble data so that the data cannot be read without first decoding it. Data encryption applies to both data in motion (during transmission) and data at rest (stored). HIPAA security provisions require technical safeguards, which include the use of encryption to protect the security and confidentiality of information that is transmitted via networks or communication systems that are public. The data are stored and transmitted in unreadable characters and symbols rather than standard text and are intended to avoid access by sniffers and hackers. Both data and passwords may be encrypted to provide further protection. Data transmission (such as in emails) that is unencrypted may result in data breaches, so secure methods of communication must be ensured for mobile devices as well as inhouse IT equipment. Data used for research may be de-identified (identifying information removed), but this is distinct from encryption.

High- and Low-Fidelity Simulations

High-fidelity simulations are those that use real or realistic equipment and materials as part of learning. This can include electroencephalogram machines, mannequins, or specialized equipment used in the work environment, so that learners can actually practice the tasks or procedures that they will carry out as part of their job. High-fidelity simulations are often the most helpful for the learner but are also the costliest because equipment may need to be dedicated for learner use. Additionally, training that involves practice and assessment of performance is often more time-consuming.

Low-fidelity simulations rely on verbal, print, video, or audio descriptions and often involve discussion of potential actions rather than actual practice. Thus, learners may be presented with a case study or scenario with specific problems and asked to describe the process for dealing with the problems. Low-fidelity simulations are less expensive and can usually be completed more quickly, but evaluation may not adequately measure clinical expertise.

Virtual Reality

Virtual reality involves participation in computer-simulated environments in which the participant often has an avatar, a visual representation of the person. Virtual-reality systems may be only viewed on the screen or may require use of special equipment, such as a wired glove or special stereoscopic goggles. Tactile information (force feedback) is also available in some applications, such as those used in medicine. The virtual reality simulation allows the person to interact and have a life-like experience in a learning environment. Virtual reality may be used to practice medical techniques, such as dissection or insertion of intravenous lines or catheters. Virtual reality systems are also used as part of therapy in some instances, such as for treatment of phobias. Second Life is a virtual online world that has been incorporated into health care educational programs, allowing students to interact in medical communities. For example, the Centers for Disease Control (CDC) have a Second Life site that provides information to "visitors" about the CDC.

Informatics Nursing Practice Test

1. If the informatics nurse is concerned that a computer system may not function well during peak times of access, the type of testing needed is:
    a. load/volume testing.
    b. system integration testing.
    c. black box testing.
    d. functional testing.

2. In preparation for the workflow redesign necessitated for implementation of an EHR, the first step should be to:
    a. conduct surveys about workflow.
    b. map the current workflow.
    c. assess the EHR requirements.
    d. assess compatibility with EHR.

3. Which resource for evidence-based research is provided by the National Library of Medicine?
    a. BMJ Publishing
    b. CINAHL
    c. PubMed
    d. *World View on Evidence-Based Nursing*

4. When considering transitioning to cloud storage and assessing vendors, the most critical assessment relates to:
    a. cost analysis.
    b. monitoring mechanisms.
    c. interoperability.
    d. regulatory compliance.

5. When utilizing a prioritization matrix to prioritize activities as a project manager, the informatics nurse must first establish:
    a. criteria and timeframe.
    b. criteria and rating scale.
    c. rating scale and timeframe.
    d. rating scale and categories.

6. An advantage of an identity and access management (IAM) system is that the IAM system:
    a. provides HIPAA-required encryption for PHI.
    b. satisfies the Code of Federal Regulations Title 21, Part 11.
    c. meets HIPAA's Security Rule requirements regarding access to PHI.
    d. meets HIPAA's Privacy Rule requirements regarding identification.

7. Which of the following standardized nursing terminologies is comprised of (1) a problem classification scheme, (2) an intervention scheme, and (3) a problem rating scale for outcomes?
    a. OMAHA
    b. NANDA-I
    c. PNDS
    d. ICNP

8. The smallest possible piece of data utilized in computer processing is the:
   a. nibble.
   b. byte.
   c. zettabyte.
   d. bit.

9. Which of the following types of software is responsible for storage management?
   a. Operating system
   b. Productivity
   c. Creativity
   d. Communication

10. Communication software is most commonly used for:
   a. documents.
   b. audio files.
   c. e-mail and IM.
   d. video files.

11. The network that connects the departments in an organization is likely a(n):
   a. VSN.
   b. LAN.
   c. WAN.
   d. MAN.

12. When an institution is transitioning to a CPOE, a primary role of the informatics nurse is that of:
   a. system designer.
   b. purchasing agent.
   c. software modifier.
   d. liaison.

13. The field of science that attempts to create intelligent technologies and then apply these technologies to the field of informatics is:
   a. cognitive science.
   b. cognitive informatics.
   c. artificial intelligence.
   d. information science.

14. In an EHR with CPOE and CDS, allergy alerts should be triggered:
   a. on physician request by accessing a link.
   b. before orders are written.
   c. after orders are written.
   d. in response to contraindicated drug orders.

15. The human-technology interface (HTI):
   a. allows user interaction with technology.
   b. standardizes applications utilized in all devices.
   c. allows access to the technology only to authorized people.
   d. connects a user device to the internet.

16. According to Peplau's Interpersonal Relations Model of nursing, the nurse-patient relationship goes through overlapping phases that include orientation, problem identification, explanation of potential solutions, and:
    a. problem evaluation.
    b. patient recovery.
    c. nurse-patient collaboration.
    d. problem resolution.

17. The nursing theory that focuses on how people react to stress through mechanisms of defense and resistance is:
    a. Total-Person Systems Model (Neuman).
    b. General Theory of Nursing (Orem).
    c. Science of Unitary Beings (Rogers).
    d. Nursing Process Theory (Orlando)

18. According to the Accelerated Rapid-Cycle Change approach to changes in healthcare, the goal is generally to:
    a. avoid responding too quickly to rapid changes.
    b. develop strategies that promote changes in health behavior.
    c. focus on the value of collaboration in achieving changes.
    d. modify and accelerate methods to respond rapidly.

19. The father of information theory and the digital age is considered to be:
    a. Albert Bandura.
    b. Alan Turing.
    c. Claude Shannon.
    d. Kurt Lewin.

20. Considering system configuration, the purpose of a mapping table is to:
    a. show the physical location of all devices that are hard-wired and network attached.
    b. outline the different types of devices (hard-wired and mobile) used in the system.
    c. plan placement of system equipment throughout an organization.
    d. provide a flow sheet to show how information flows through the system.

21. When evaluating staff members' readiness to learn in preparation for training, the 4 factors to consider include (1) physical factors, (2) knowledge/education, (3) psychological/emotional status, and (4):
    a. security.
    b. experience.
    c. investment.
    d. determination.

22. Which type of system would be most efficient to track the movement of equipment through the hospital?
    a. Barcode
    b. Closed circuit TV
    c. Passive radio frequency identification (pRFI)
    d. Active radio frequency identification (aRFI)

23. Incentives for "meaningful use" of EHRs are provided by:
 a. CMS.
 b. NIH.
 c. FDA.
 d. FCC.

24. The purpose of the NDNQI is to:
 a. use nursing-sensitive indicators to determine accountability.
 b. provide a guide for collection of data.
 c. collect nursing-sensitive indicators from participating hospitals.
 d. carry out predictive analysis based on nursing-sensitive indicators.

25. A hospital survey of nurses and clinicians showed that 88% used their smartphones for some work-related activity, such as looking up information or texting patient information. The best solution is to:
 a. prohibit all smartphones in the work environment.
 b. develop an acceptable use policy for personal devices.
 c. advise staff to avoid breaching patient confidentiality.
 d. provide hospital-owned smartphones to all staff.

26. Stage 2 of the meaningful use criteria regarding adoption of standardized terminology includes use of which of the following for procedures?
 a. SNOMED-CT
 b. LOINC
 c. CPT
 d. ICD 9/10

27. The area of informatics that is most invested in assisting patients to utilize health-enabling technologies to prevent, monitor, and manage disease is:
 a. public health informatics.
 b. consumer health informatics.
 c. translational bioinformatics.
 d. clinical informatics.

28. From the clinical nurse's perspective, NANDA-I is generally found to be most useful for:
 a. planning care of patients.
 b. ensuring appropriate outcomes.
 c. retrieving information about disease.
 d. providing appropriate interventions.

29. The business concept of "planned obsolescence" is utilized in the field of technology primarily to:
 a. ensure organizations modernize.
 b. prevent loss of functionality.
 c. comply with regulatory requirements.
 d. ensure market demand continues.

30. Workflow design regarding patient care requires input primarily from:
    a. informatics nurses.
    b. IT personnel.
    c. clinicians and nurses.
    d. vendor engineers.

31. When planning for transition to an EHR and training needs, the informatics nurse is concerned that staff members lack necessary technological skills. The best method to assess this is probably:
    a. gap analysis.
    b. SWOT analysis.
    c. surveys.
    d. interviews.

32. In a relational database, "redundancy" refers to:
    a. data that provide no valuable information.
    b. backup of data in a second hosting site.
    c. duplication of attribute data.
    d. backup methods of accessing data.

33. The structure of data supported by a hierarchical database is:
    a. many to many.
    b. one to many.
    c. many to one.
    d. one to many and many to one.

34. The primary disadvantage to an alert that requires manual activation for viewing is that:
    a. activating the alert requires too much time.
    b. activating the alert distracts healthcare providers.
    c. alerts requiring activation are of little value.
    d. healthcare providers may not activate the alert.

35. When utilizing SAS Enterprise guide to query a database, if the derived data are to be saved permanently, the correct format is:
    a. data view.
    b. report.
    c. data table.
    d. data table or data view.

36. If an input device is connected to the system but the system does not recognize the device, the device is in the state of:
    a. undefined.
    b. defined.
    c. available.
    d. unavailable.

37. The type of information system report that contains data about the system, hardware, software, workstations, and servers is:
    a. informational.
    b. error/exception.
    c. baseline.
    d. configuration.

38. The ethical principle that is most represented in the AMIA Code of Ethics (principles of professional and ethical conduct for AMIA members) is:
    a. non-malfeasance.
    b. beneficence.
    c. justice.
    d. autonomy.

39. During the phase of technical development, a constructive assessment of the cognitive aspects could evaluate the response to:
    a. the effort needed to document in the EHR while interviewing a patient.
    b. the number of screens the user must access to transfer a patient.
    c. the number of mouse clicks needed to complete an activity.
    d. the eye strain from looking at a screen for prolonged periods.

40. When conducting technical verifications to determine if a system should become operational, the most difficult assessment is usually of:
    a. capacity.
    b. security.
    c. interoperability.
    d. software installation.

41. During observational testing for the adaptation phase of an information system, the informatics nurse observes users taking notes of data to enter into the system later when they have more time. This suggests a(n):
    a. cognitive problem.
    b. compliance problem.
    c. training problem.
    d. ergonomic problem.

42. Which of the following represents the purpose of a functionality assessment of an information system?
    a. To determine if users are able to navigate the interface
    b. To determine if the system responds as intended
    c. To determine if the system complies with the work processes
    d. To determine if the system demonstrates adequate interoperability

43. During the explorative phase of selecting an information system, which of the following assessment methods is most useful in order to observe the practices in an organization and to identify those agents controlling change?
    a. Field study
    b. Focus group
    c. SWOT analysis
    d. Delphi

44. According to the HL7 group, the three different types of interoperability are:
    a. functional, ergonomic, and cognitive.
    b. technical, semantic, and process/social.
    c. technical, interactive, and non-interactive.
    d. functional, technical, and ergonomic.

45. Which of the following segments of the National Drug Code (NDC) format for barcoding medications is assigned by the FDA?
    a. Product code
    b. Package code
    c. Product and package code
    d. Labeler code

46. HL7 CDA is a standard utilized for:
    a. document exchange.
    b. security provisions.
    c. data mining.
    d. data warehousing.

47. A primary advantage of using coded data over free text is that coded data:
    a. allow for fuller description.
    b. are more flexible.
    c. ensure consistency/standardized vocabulary.
    d. eliminate errors.

48. The agency/organization that develops standards for information systems to support documentation of nursing practice is:
    a. ANSI.
    b. HL7.
    c. CMS.
    d. ANA.

49. When assessing compliance for the EHR with CPOE CDS system, the informatics nurse notes that alerts are frequent and disruptive, resulting in hard stops, and they are routinely overridden or ignored. The best solution is probably to:
    a. eliminate non-critical alerts.
    b. eliminate hard stops.
    c. implement tiered alerts.
    d. provide additional training.

50. Which of the following is a data element set utilized for nursing administration?
    a. NMDS
    b. NMMDS
    c. PNDS
    d. PCDS

51. Which of the following is a CDS intervention that targets preventive care?
    a. A recommendation for immunization
    b. A list of possible diagnoses associated with patient symptoms
    c. Reminders for drug interactions
    d. An alert that prescribed medication is not in the formulary

52. If the CDS system recommends a therapy that the clinician ignores, the system usually:
    a. sends an alert to administration.
    b. locks down until the action is taken.
    c. takes no further action.
    d. sends repeated alerts about the therapy.

53. In terms of information, "longevity" refers to information being:
    a. useful for a variety of different purposes.
    b. available at any location.
    c. easily accessible.
    d. usable beyond the current clinical situation.

54. According to the International Technical Standard ISO 18104:2003, for a nursing action to be valid it must include at least:
    a. focus and judgment.
    b. action and target.
    c. focus and target.
    d. action and judgment.

55. If developing a chart to display data about the age distribution of patients admitted to the oncology department over a one-month period, a useful type of graphic display would be a:
    a. scattergram.
    b. pie chart.
    c. digital dashboard.
    d. balanced scorecard.

56. Considering ethical implications for data dissemination, data that contain ID codes that are linked to names, which are not divulged, would be classified as:
    a. de-identified.
    b. potentially identifiable.
    c. identifiable.
    d. anonymous.

57. Which governmental agency is responsible for oversight and enforcement of HIPAA's Privacy Rule?
    a. Centers for Disease Control and Prevention (CDC)
    b. Federal Communications Commission (FCC)
    c. Food and Drug Administration (FDA)
    d. Office for Civil Rights (OCR)

58. When integrating data analysis into the performance improvement process, the model of integration that includes developing multidisciplinary teams that function in different areas but all report to the same project manager is:
    a. organizational.
    b. functional/coordinated.
    c. functional/integrated.
    d. departmental.

59. If the informatics nurse provides computers and a test version of software for staff nurses to use during training, this would be classified as:
    a. low fidelity simulation.
    b. high fidelity simulation.
    c. virtual reality.
    d. modeling.

60. The type of component suitability testing that determines whether or not an input produces the correct output by using test cases is:
    a. operational system.
    b. defense building.
    c. fault injection.
    d. black box.

61. The technical standard that applies to accessibility of software is:
    a. ISO 900:2008.
    b. ISO 9241-171:2008.
    c. ISO/IEC 27001:2013.
    d. ISO 639-4:2010.

62. Which of the following technologies encodes audio files into digital files that can be streamed over the internet?
    a. Wi-Fi
    b. Bluetooth
    c. VoIP
    d. NFC

63. For archiving data, federal regulations require that clinical health records of living adults be maintained for at least:
    a. 2 years.
    b. 6 years.
    c. 10 years.
    d. 18 years.

64. A primary advantage of tiered archival storage is:
    a. cost effectiveness.
    b. faster access.
    c. decreased management needs.
    d. compliance with the FDA approval process for image storage.

65. Which of the following domain suffixes is likely to deliver the most reliable information?
    a. .com
    b. .org
    c. .gov
    d. .edu

66. The goal of translational research is to:
    a. decrease variability in nursing practice.
    b. search coded data for patterns.
    c. translate foreign healthcare articles into English.
    d. translate medical/nursing research into interventions.

67. In an evidence hierarchy, the type of evidence that would have the highest priority is:
    a. meta-analysis.
    b. individual experimental studies.
    c. nonexperimental studies.
    d. expert opinion.

68. When planning staff training for EHR implementation, the informatics nurse should keep in mind that the best retention is likely to occur if the participants:
    a. read material about EHRs.
    b. listen to a lecture and audiotapes about EHRs.
    c. research and give presentations about EHRs.
    d. practice using the EHR with real equipment.

69. Considering the systems in a healthcare organization, a suprasystem would include:
    a. external agencies.
    b. staff members.
    c. patients.
    d. rules and regulations.

70. If the informatics nurse wants to make training materials available in audio and video format for staff members, the best method is probably to:
    a. set up viewing/listening inservice meetings.
    b. provide viewing/listening in staff lounges/cafeteria.
    c. provide downloadable digital materials.
    d. sign out DVDs to staff members.

71. If a hospital develops a social media site to provide informational content to consumers but finds that it has almost no traffic, the best solution is to:
    a. add more content to the site.
    b. conduct surveys and reevaluate.
    c. take down the site.
    d. hire an expert to create a new site.

72. As project manager, the informatics nurse has encountered a team member who talks compulsively during meetings and ignores suggestions that all team members participate. The best solution is to:
   a. remove the person from the team so that it can be more effective.
   b. confront the person during the meeting.
   c. discuss the problem face-to-face outside of the meeting.
   d. refer the person to the Human Resources Department for counseling.

73. When sending a reminder of a team meeting by E-mail, the most important information to include in the E-mail is:
   a. purpose and agenda.
   b. names of participants.
   c. list of outcomes goals.
   d. a reminder about the responsibility to attend.

74. If the information programmed in a CDS system is incorrect and a patient suffers harm because of this, the person responsible for the incorrect information may be accused of:
   a. negligent misstatement.
   b. gross negligence.
   c. negligence.
   d. malpractice.

75. According to Ruesch, the five major elements that are required for communication are (1) sender, (2) message, (3) receiver, (4) feedback, and (5):
   a. content.
   b. motivation.
   c. purpose.
   d. context.

76. With Total Quality Management (TQM), the primary focus is on:
   a. providing cost-effective care.
   b. satisfying the needs of the customers.
   c. ensuring organizational consistency.
   d. promoting staff satisfaction.

77. The Quality and Safety Education for Nurses (QSEN) project's informatics competency includes the 3 elements of:
   a. knowledge, skills, and attitude.
   b. data, information, and knowledge.
   c. data collection, data storage, and data safety.
   d. safety, privacy, and utilization.

78. When carrying out an SQL query of a relational database, which of the following is classified as a *logical* operator?
   a. %
   b. <>
   c. BETWEEN
   d. *

79. If the informatics nurse has found a new application that may enhance the existing EHR with CPOE CDS system, the first concern before recommending the application is:
    a. cost.
    b. compatibility.
    c. usability.
    d. safety.

80. An example of "web surfing" is:
    a. using a search engine, such as Google, to obtain links.
    b. using a Boolean search of a database to obtain articles.
    c. using SQL to obtain data from a relational database.
    d. navigating the internet by clicking links for one site to another.

81. With encryption of data, "stickiness" refers to:
    a. a high level of encryption.
    b. the degree to which encryption persists when encrypted data are moved.
    c. the ability of encryption software to encrypt different types of data.
    d. utilization of the same key to both encrypt and decrypt.

82. When decommissioning a computer information system (CIS), one of the purposes of the Records Management Plan (RMP) is to:
    a. ensure disposition of data corresponds to federal/state regulations.
    b. identify activities/tasks associated with shutdown of the system.
    c. identify components of the budget that must be transitioned.
    d. identify contractual obligations in relation to termination.

83. Which of the following is an example of a qualitative approach to obtaining user feedback about a computer information system?
    a. Obtaining error rates from the database
    b. Surveying with a ranking scale
    c. Obtaining usage rates from the database
    d. Conducting a one-on-one interview

84. In the three-phase change management process (Prosci), which of the following activities is part of phase I, preparing for change?
    a. Develop plans for change management
    b. Identify and manage resistance to change
    c. Define the strategy for managing change
    d. Implement change management plans

85. When completing process mapping for workflow, which of the following is an example of a process at the micro level?
    a. Admission procedures
    b. Transferring a patient from one unit to another
    c. Completing a blood draw for a lab test
    d. Completing wound assessment, irrigation, and dressing change

86. At what point in implementation of an EHR should a chart migration plan be formulated?
    a. Before going live
    b. Before purchase of an EHR
    c. During the transition to live
    d. After going live

87. The GUI serves to:
    a. ensure that the operating system functions correctly.
    b. facilitate interaction between the user and the computer.
    c. coordinate use of input and output devices.
    d. provide security for the operating system of the computer.

88. When implementing an EHR, many paper patient documents were scanned into the new system rather than coded. The primary disadvantage to this is that the data:
    a. are harder to access.
    b. are in two formats.
    c. may be corrupted.
    d. cannot be mined.

89. As part of the American Recovery and Reinvestment Act (ARRA), the Office of the National Coordinator for Health Information Technology (ONC) established 62 Regional Extension Centers (RECs), whose purpose is to:
    a. assist healthcare organizations to adopt EHRs.
    b. ensure compliance with Meaningful Use requirements.
    c. monitor organizations that have implemented EHRs.
    d. conduct research utilizing data mining of health records.

90. When notified that a costly upgrade to the EHR is scheduled for implementation within the next few months, the first step should be to:
    a. evaluate the need for the upgrade.
    b. send RFIs to other vendors.
    c. determine how long the current version will be supported.
    d. request details and a demonstration.

91. When the informatics nurse notes that there has been a marked increase in help-desk tickets to one hospital unit, the first action should be to:
    a. provide additional training for the unit staff.
    b. interview the staff on the unit.
    c. analyze the types of help-desk tickets.
    d. interview help desk staff members.

92. An example of aggregate data is:
    a. a laboratory report.
    b. hospital census data for the state.
    c. a patient consent form.
    d. a patient treatment plan.

93. When considering improvements to workflow processes, the first issue to address is whether steps in a process:
   a. can be combined.
   b. should be increased.
   c. require alternate paths.
   d. can be eliminated.

94. If the hospital is considering a telemedicine venture that would provide internet consultation and treatment to rural patients in four states, the first concern is:
   a. licensure.
   b. security.
   c. patient access.
   d. patient-physician relationships.

95. Considering cloud architecture, if software applications are hosted by the vendor and then distributed to the organization via the internet, this model is referred to as:
   a. platform as a service (PaaS).
   b. infrastructure as a service (IaaS).
   c. software as a service (SAS).
   d. storage as a service (SAS).

96. If an institution permits personalized order sets for the CPOE CDS system because of a specialized treatment center, the order sets should be reviewed at least:
   a. monthly.
   b. biannually.
   c. biennially.
   d. annually.

97. In an EHR, orderable items, such as radiology tests and medications, should be requested by:
   a. conducting a free text search.
   b. browsing through an alphabetical listing.
   c. querying with a Boolean search.
   d. sending an interdepartmental message.

98. If laboratory results input into the EHR show critical values, the clinician should be:
   a. provided an alert within the EHR.
   b. sent a text message.
   c. notified verbally if there is no response in two hours.
   d. notified verbally immediately.

99. A collection of data about one particular hospital unit to facilitate decision-making by administration is a:
   a. data mart.
   b. data warehouse.
   c. data file.
   d. data mine.

100. As a project manager who is charged with creating a number of teams to facilitate transition to an EHR, the informatics nurse should limit team size to:
    a. <4 members.
    b. <6 members.
    c. <10 members.
    d. <15 members.

101. When displaying patient data for clinical decision-making, which type of display tends to slow cognitive processing of the data?
    a. Line graph.
    b. Table.
    c. Pictorial displays.
    d. Multiple displays on one screen.

102. According to systems theory (von Bertalanffy), the element of a system that comprises actions that take place in order to transform input is:
    a. Throughput.
    b. Output.
    c. Evaluation.
    d. Feedback.

103. The type of personal health record (PHR) that is standalone and not connected to a particular system or electronic health record (EHR) is:
    a. Paper/Personal files.
    b. Untethered.
    c. Tethered.
    d. Networked.

104. The type of data that includes pharmacy transactions, required reports, financial information, and demographic information is:
    a. Medical/Clinical.
    b. Knowledge based.
    c. Comparison
    d. Aggregate.

105. The most commonly used structured query language (SQL) operation is:
    a. Clause.
    b. Expression.
    c. Query.
    d. Predicate.

106. According to Part I of the International Medical Informatics Association (IMIA) Code of Ethics, legitimate infringement refers to:
    a. Consideration for the greater good of society in regard to an individual's right to privacy.
    b. Consideration of the rules of conduct related to the right to privacy.
    c. Maintenance of an individual's right to privacy.
    d. Right to access of personal information.

107. In Kurt Lewin's change theory, the first stage, motivation to change, is also referred to as:
    a. Freezing.
    b. Unfreezing.
    c. Unfrozen.
    d. Refreezing.

108. When conducting a usability study to compare new practice with older practice, an essential component is:
    a. Asking users to assign usability ratings.
    b. Focusing on one aspect of use.
    c. Administering questionnaires to assess satisfaction.
    d. Determining measures of equivalency.

109. The method used to determine monetary savings resulting from planned interventions is:
    a. Cost-benefit analysis.
    b. Cost-effective analysis.
    c. Efficacy study.
    d. Cost-utility analysis.

110. The data representation method that can be used across multiple platforms to represent text for most languages, including Asian, is:
    a. Binary code.
    b. Hexadecimal code.
    c. Unicode Standard code.
    d. Extended binary coded decimal interchange code.

111. Allowing other health care professionals to view an authorized password most often results in which type of patient data misuse?
    a. Identity theft.
    b. Unauthorized access.
    c. Dissemination of private information.
    d. Security breach.

112. The primary purpose of sending a request for information (RFI) to multiple vendors is to:
    a. Aid in the elimination and selection process.
    b. Meet regulatory requirements.
    c. Eliminate the need for a request for quote (RFQ).
    d. Complete a cost-utility analysis.

113. Bloom's taxonomy outlines behaviors necessary for learning. Which 3 kinds of learning does the theory describe?
    a. Auditory, visual, and kinesthetic.
    b. Formal and informal.
    c. Attitudes, subjective norms, and behavioral intention.
    d. Cognitive, affective, and psychomotor.

114. Using Boolean logic for a query, which of the following would pull up articles about wound care that involved the use of povidone-iodine without antibiotics?
  a. Wound AND povidone-iodine.
  b. Wound NOT antibiotics.
  c. Wound AND povidone-iodine NOT antibiotics.
  d. Wound OR povidone-iodine OR antibiotics.

115. The first step to knowledge discovery in databases (KDD) is:
  a. data mining.
  b. data selection.
  c. preprocessing data.
  d. transforming data.

116. The Health Insurance Portability and Accountability Act (HIPAA) mandates privacy and security rules (CFR, Title 45, Part 164) to ensure that health information and individual privacy is protected. Which of the following is part of the privacy rules?
  a. Protected information includes conversations between a doctor and other health care providers.
  b. Any health information must be secure and protected against threats, hazards, or nonpermitted disclosure.
  c. Implementation specifications must be addressed for any adopted standards.
  d. Access controls must include unique identifier.

117. Which of the following processes is most useful in determining the steps required to move from a current state of performance to a new one, including the need for actions and resources?
  a. Cost-benefit analysis.
  b. Gap analysis.
  c. Outcomes analysis.
  d. Return on investment (ROI) analysis.

118. Detecting anomalies, identifying relationships, classifying, regressing, and summarizing are steps to:
  a. Data aggregation.
  b. Data representation.
  c. Data fusion.
  d. Data mining.

119. The primary advantage of Voice-over-Internet Protocol (VoIP) devices over landline telephones is:
  a. Speed of transmission.
  b. Cost saving.
  c. Ease of use.
  d. End-user acceptance.

120. The nursing theory that includes the concepts of self-care, self-care deficit, and nursing systems is:
  a. the general theory of nursing (Orem).
  b. the total-person systems models (Neuman).
  c. nursing process theory (Orlando).
  d. the crisis theory (Hoff).

121. The messaging standard primarily utilized to communicate clinical data is:
  a. American Society for Testing and Materials (ASTM).
  b. Institute of Electrical and Electronics Engineers (IEEE)
  c. Health Level 7 (HL7).
  d. Digital Imaging and Communications in Medicine (DICOM).

122. In terms of communication devices for networks, the purpose of a hub is to:
  a. Bring network data together.
  b. Connect networks at the data link level.
  c. Determine data's destination.
  d. Send data to the correct destination.

123. According to the Health Information Technology for Economic and Clinical Health Act (HITECH) security provisions, a breach in security of personal health information requires notification of:
  a. Administration.
  b. Physician.
  c. US Department of Health and Human Services (HHS).
  d. Individuals impacted and US Department of Health and Human Services (HHS).

124. Which of the following is an example of a disconnected token?
  a. Smart card.
  b. Radio frequency identification (RFID) device.
  c. Personal identification number (PIN).
  d. USB token.

125. In Claude Shannon's information theory, channel capacity is:
  a. the ratio between a signal's magnitude and interfering "noise" magnitude.
  b. the amount of energy, code or bits, required to communicate or store one symbol in the communication process.
  c. the determining factor in the amount of information that can be transmitted with the smallest rate of error.
  d. the ability to encode a message utilizing code or bits.

126. According to the Theory of Cognitive Dissonance (Festinger), which of the following is most likely to change if dissonance occurs?
  a. Beliefs
  b. Behaviors
  c. Actions
  d. Emotions

127. Data definitions must be based on a solid understanding of statistical analysis and epidemiological concepts. Specific issues that must be addressed include sensitivity, which means that data should:

    a. measure the target adequately so that the results have predictive value.

    b. be classified according to subsets, taking variables into consideration.

    c. include only those cases specific to the needs of the measurement and exclude those that may be similar but are a different population, decreasing the number of false positives.

    d. include all positive cases, taking into account variables, decreasing the number of false negatives.

128. An easy to access and read computer program that integrates a variety of performance measures or key indicators into one display to provide an overview of an organization is referred to as a:

    a. scattergram.

    b. dashboard.

    c. balanced scorecard.

    d. histogram.

129. For ease of reading, when highlighting text on the screen, the best method is to:

    a. italicize.

    b. bold.

    c. underline.

    d. place text on a colored background.

130. An essential component of a cognitive walkthrough when assessing usability is:

    a. exit questionnaire.

    b. pre-assessment interview.

    c. observational note taking.

    d. "think aloud" procedure.

131. User-acceptance testing (UAT) should begin with:

    a. designing the testing plan and test cases, considering risks and the skills of the end-users.

    b. analyzing the basic requirements of the system and the organization.

    c. identifying the end-user acceptance scenarios.

    d. describing a testing plan, including different severity levels based on real-world conditions.

132. According to the human-computer interaction (HCI) framework (Staggers), the primary focus of HCI is:

    a. usability.

    b. design.

    c. efficiency of operations.

    d. interoperability.

133. The correct elbow angle for a person when sitting in a chair and using a computer keyboard is:

    a. 45 degrees.

    b. 60 degrees.

    c. 90 degrees.

    d. 120 degrees.

134. The communication theory that describes communication as an exchange system in which people attempt to negotiate a return on their "investment" in much the same way that people engage in commerce is:
    a. Social Penetration Theory (Altman and Taylor).
    b. Communication Accommodation Theory (Giles).
    c. Spiral of Silence Theory (Noelle-Neuman).
    d. Social Exchange Theory (Homans, Thibaut, and Kelley).

135. When determining the burden of proof for acts of negligence, risk management would classify willfully providing inadequate care while disregarding the safety and security of another as:
    a. negligent conduct.
    b. gross negligence.
    c. contributory negligence.
    d. comparative negligence.

136. An important element of a personal health record (PHR) is:
    a. accessibility from specific sites.
    b. information derived from primary physicians only.
    c. disclosure of who has entered data and accessed data.
    d. health information beginning with adulthood.

137. In order to participate in the Centers for Medicare and Medicaid Services (CMS) Medicare incentive program for adoption of electronic health records, those applying must demonstrate that they:
    a. use certified EHR systems that have demonstrated they can store and share patient data securely, maintaining privacy.
    b. have a 5-year plan in place for transition to the EHR.
    c. will begin participation by 2020.
    d. participate in a Regional Health Improvement Plan (RHIP).

138. In trending analysis, a sentinel event is indicated by a:
    a. run.
    b. trend.
    c. astronomical value.
    d. cycle.

139. Leapfrog Safe Practices score is used as a basis for:
    a. promoting evidence-based practice through funding of 14 Evidence-based Practice Centers (EPCs).
    b. providing collaborative training within the network related to safe clinical practice.
    c. providing fellowships to help professionals gain experience and expertise in health-related fields.
    d. assessing the progress a health care organization is making on 30 safe practices.

140. The National Quality Forum's safe practices specifically regarding managing medications include:
    a. documenting care properly.
    b. implementing a computerized prescriber order entry (CPOE) system.
    c. informing patients of risks.
    d. providing discharge planning.

141. When an input device is connected to a system the information of the device is present in the database and configured to the operating system, the state of the device is classified as:
    a. undefined.
    b. defined.
    c. available.
    d. not available/stopped.

142. Simulations that rely on verbal, print, video, or audio descriptions are classified as:
    a. functional.
    b. process.
    c. low fidelity.
    d. high fidelity.

143. When generating a report of an information system, an error/exception report can indicate:
    a. data about the system itself.
    b. data outside of normal parameters.
    c. changes occurring over a period of time.
    d. how the elements of the system compare to the baseline.

144. In over-the-shoulder instruction, most instruction is per:
    a. demonstration.
    b. group interaction.
    c. lecture.
    d. computer-assisted instruction (CAI).

145. New policies are being instituted, based on evidence-based research, but some staff members are vocally resistant to the changes. What is the most appropriate action?
    a. Advise staff that complaining is counterproductive
    b. Provide honest information about the reasons for the changes and how the changes will affect staff
    c. Suggest that staff vote on whether to implement the changes
    d. File a report with human resources about those complaining

146. The teaching model in which learning takes place outside of a formal classroom with materials provided or recommended by the instructor is:
    a. guided focus.
    b. independent study.
    c. cognitive apprenticeship.
    d. cooperative.

147. In a process diagram, such as a clinical workflow chart, the parallelogram is typically used to indicate:
    a. connectors with diverging paths with multiple arrows coming in but only one going out.
    b. conditional decision (Yes/No or True/False).
    c. direction of flow.
    d. input and output (Start/End).

148. In a database, the type of data that is usually used to represent the count of something is:
     a. categorical.
     b. quantitative.
     c. discrete.
     d. continuous.

149. Which of the following is true about current procedural terminology (CPT) codes?
     a. They were developed by the World Health Organization
     b. The used to code for medical and surgical treatments, diagnostics, and procedures
     c. They used to code for diagnosis
     d. They are consistent with *DSM-5*, cancer registry codes, and nursing classifications

150. Under provisions of the Americans with Disabilities Act (ADA) (1992), employers are allowed to ask applicants if they:
     a. need work accommodations.
     b. have any type of disability.
     c. can carry out incidental functions of the job.
     d. will consent to a medical examination prior to a job offer.

Answer Key and Explanations

1. A: If the informatics nurse is concerned that a computer system may not function well during peak times of access, the type of testing needed is load/volume testing. This is a non-functional testing for reliability that assesses the ability of the system to function under various loads, such as at peak times when multiple users in multiple departments are accessing the system. The purpose of load/volume testing is to determine the maximum load capacity and to identify the load at which problems begin to occur. Testing is done at both the safe working load (SWL) and above the SWL.

2. B: In preparation for the workflow redesign necessitated for implementation of an EHR, the first step should be to map the current workflow at the macro, mini, and micro levels, focusing on areas that are likely to be most impacted by the implementation. Examples of affected areas include patient admission and discharge, laboratory and medication orders, scheduling appointments, referrals, and billing for services.

3. C: PubMed is a resource for evidence-based research that is provided by the National Library of Medicine, which was developed by the National Center for Biotechnology Information (NCBI). PubMed provides access to numerous databases with 24 million citations from MEDLINE (the National Library of Medicine's bibliographic database with references to life sciences and biomedical sciences), life science journals, and electronic books with links to full text when it is available.

4. D: When considering transitioning to cloud storage and assessing vendors, the most critical assessment relates to compliance with regulatory requirements because if the vendor cannot verify that the company meets HIPAA requirements and satisfies the Code of Federal Regulations Title 21, Part 11 (which provides regulations regarding electronic records and electronic signatures), then security of patient data may be inadequate. Other important considerations include cost analysis (including cost of implementation and ongoing costs), monitoring mechanisms, and interoperability.

5. B: When utilizing a prioritization matrix to prioritize projects as a project manager, the informatics nurse must first establish criteria and a rating scale. The criteria include those factors that are utilized to determine how important each project is; for example, a project mandated by regulations is more important than a project that may improve customer satisfaction. A rating scale for each project should be established with numeric values (such as 1 to 10) used to demonstrate how effective the project is in meeting the criteria. A typical prioritization matrix may have up to a dozen criteria.

6. C: An advantage of an identity and access management (IAM) system is that the IAM system meets HIPAA's Security Rule requirements regarding access to PHI through identity management. An IAM system provides, captures, updates, and records user IDs and provides appropriate access privileges, preventing "privilege creep," which increases risks to security. The IAM system should provide authentication (single sign-in and session management), authorization (based on roles, rules, and attributes), user management (provisioning and password management), and a central directory.

7. A: OMAHA is standardized nursing terminology that is comprised of (1) a problem classification scheme, (2) an intervention scheme, and (3) a problem rating scale for outcome. OMAHA was developed by the Visiting Nurse Association in Omaha, Nebraska, in the 1970s and was later

developed further through research projects funded by the US Department of Health and Human Services. OMAHA is in the public domain but must be used as published (as opposed to modified).

8. D: The smallest piece of data utilized in computer processing is the bit (binary digit), which comprises zeros (off) and ones (on). Four bits equal one nibble, eight bits equal one byte, 1024 bytes equal one kilobyte, 1024 kilobytes equal one megabyte, and 1024 megabytes equal one gigabyte. (Note that these measurements are often rounded down to 1000). Bits are used to describe transmission speed and bytes are used to describe storage, so there may be some confusion regarding the terms.

9. A: Operating system software is responsible for storage management. Operating software, which loads first when the computer is turned on, is the most critical, handling both hardware and software applications, and is responsible for a number of processes, including management of memory, devices, processors, application interface, and the user interface. Operating systems include Mac OS X, Unix, Linux, and Microsoft Windows. Current operating systems generally support multiple users and they can also multi-task, so that users can work in more than one application at a time.

10. C: Communication software is most commonly used for e-mail and IM (instant messaging) to allow users to communicate easily with each other and may include conferencing software that is used for virtual meetings. Documents are usually created utilizing productive software, such as Microsoft Office, which includes Word and Excel. Desktop publishing applications, such as Adobe InDesign, are also forms of productive software. Audio and video files are usually created utilizing creative software, such as Apple QuickTime and Real Studio.

11. B: The network that connects the departments in an organization is likely a LAN (local-area network). Many LANs nowadays are Wi-Fi-based: WLANs (wireless local area networks). Larger networks, such as in a city or an area of a city are MANs (metropolitan area networks). A network that encompasses a much larger area, such as a country, is a WAN (wide area network). VSNs (virtual social networks) are one type of targeted network that often serve one group, such as informatics nurses, and provide the opportunity for sharing experiences and collaborating.

12. D: When an institution is transitioning to a CPOE, a primary role of the informatics nurse is that of liaison to promote multidisciplinary collaboration and cooperation among the various members of the healthcare team, including nurses, physicians, and IT specialists, to ensure that the end-product has the functionality that is needed for workflow and that it meets the requirements for safety and security. Needs regarding both hardware and software must be clearly communicated to IT personnel.

13. C: The field of science that applies intelligent technologies to the field of informatics is artificial intelligence. Researchers in artificial intelligence must engineer general intelligence and reasoning skills into the artificial intelligence programs as well as the ability to develop and learn from experiences and errors and to process natural language. One example of an artificial intelligence program is Siri, which responds to verbal queries and is found on Apple devices, such as the iPhone and iPad.

14. B: In an EHR with CPOE and CDS, allergy alerts should be triggered before orders are written and they should be automated. Alerts that occur after orders are written are more likely to be ignored or overridden. Additional alerts, including hard stops, should occur if orders for contraindicated drugs or drugs to which the patient is allergic are ordered despite the original alert.

The alerts should be carefully evaluated because excessive alerts may result in "alert fatigue" to the point that clinicians begin to ignore them.

15. A: The human-technology interface (HTI) allows user interaction with technology, so HTI may include touch (as with touch screens), keyboards, light pens, barcodes, ID badges, or voice (for voice-activated devices or applications). HTIs vary widely according to the hardware and software involved and may include various levels of security. In some cases, there is virtually no security because the interaction may be activated by simply turning on a switch. In other cases, the interaction may be predicated on the use of a user name and password or other method of identification.

16. D: According to Peplau's Interpersonal Relations Model of nursing, the nurse-patient relationship goes through overlapping phases that include orientation, problem identification, explanation of potential solutions, and problem resolution. Peplau believed that collaboration between the nurse and patient was especially important and that the nurse acts as a "maturing force" to help the patient. Peplau also stressed the importance of the patient being treated with dignity and respect and believed that a positive or negative environment could affect a patient accordingly.

17. A: The nursing theory that focuses on how people react to stress through mechanisms of defense and resistance is the Total-Person Systems Model of Betty Neuman (1972). According to this theory, stressors may be intrapersonal, interpersonal, or extrapersonal, and the nurse carries out primary (preventive steps taken before reaction to stress), secondary (facilitation of the internal ability to resist and to remove the stressor), and tertiary interventions (supportive actions) to assist the patient to stabilize and to avoid negative effects resulting from stressors.

18. D: According to the Accelerated Rapid-Cycle Change approach to changes in healthcare, the goal is generally to modify and accelerate methods in order to respond quickly, generally aiming to double or triple the rate of quality improvement. Rapid action teams (RATs) focus on finding and testing solutions rather than analysis. Team meetings and workflow are organized over 6-week periods, beginning at week one with reviewing information and clarifying opportunities for quality improvement and ending at week 6 with implementation.

19. C: In 1948, Claude Shannon, a mathematician, wrote a paper that laid out the basis for modern information theory: "A Mathematical Theory of Communication." Shannon showed how all forms of information (including text, telephone signals, video, audio, and telephone) could be encoded through a binary system of 0s and 1s and transmitted error free; he also showed how the amount of information carried over a system of communication could be calculated mathematically. Shannon demonstrated that switching circuits could be endowed with decision-making ability (applicable to artificial intelligence).

20. A: Considering system configuration, the purpose of a mapping table is to show the physical location of all devices that are hardwired and network-attached, including computer terminals, workstations, and printers. This mapping table should help to demonstrate that placement is adequate so that clinicians do not have to walk more than 50 feet to gain access to the system and that the number of devices is adequate so that wait time is minimal. Additionally, the mapping should show that printers are available within 25 feet of each acute care unit and outpatient exam room.

21. B: When evaluating staff members' readiness to learn in preparation for training, the 4 factors to consider include (1) physical factors (ability to see and hear, physical abilities/impairments, manual dexterity, pain), (2) knowledge/education (general, cognitive ability, topic-specific knowledge, general literacy, health literacy), (3) psychological/emotional status (stress, confidence, anxiety, depression, ability to cope with stress), and (4) experience (various life factors, such as cultural background, work history, and personal experiences as well as previous experience with learning).

22. D: The type of system that would be most efficient to track the movement of equipment and supplies through the hospital is active radio frequency identification (aRFI). With RFI, equipment contains embedded digital memory chips with codes unique to the piece of equipment. Sensors then receive signals from the chips. In passive RFI, signals are only transmitted when the chip is in close proximity to the sensor. However, in active RFI continuous transmission of signal between the chip and the sensor occurs, allowing more accurate tracking.

23. A: Incentives for "meaningful use" of EHRs are provided by CMS. The American Recovery and Reinvestment Act (ARRA) and its Health Information Technology Act (HITECH) provision allocated $19 billion dollars for a 5-year period for incentives for hospitals and ambulatory care centers, beginning in 2011, and authorized the CMS to provide the incentives to hospitals and eligible providers. Five criteria for meaningful use include (1) improve healthcare quality and reduce disparities, (2) engage both patients and families, (3) improve coordination of care, (4) improve population and public health, and (5) ensure PHI is secure and private.

24. C: The purpose of the National Database of Nursing Quality Indicators (NDNQI) is to collect nursing-sensitive indicators from participating hospitals and to make this collected data available to both participants and researchers who can compare data in order to establish benchmarks and use the data to improve the quality of nursing care. The data can also be used with analytic software for predictive analytics to identify patients who are at risk and who need targeted preventive interventions.

25. B: Smartphones are ubiquitous, and trying to ban them from a hospital is not practical; however, an acceptable use policy for personal devices should be developed with strict guidelines. Numerous informational applications (such as drug guides) are available for smartphones and these pose little risk, but texting a physician with a patient update may violate not only federal regulations but State Board of Nursing regulations. Most personal smartphones do not have adequate passwords or encryption or the ability to remotely destroy data if the phone is stolen or lost.

26. C: Stage 2 of the meaningful use criteria regarding adoption of standardized terminology includes use of CPT (Current Procedural Terminology) for procedures. SNOMED-CT (Systemized Nomenclatures for Medicine, Clinical Terms) is used for medical terms. LOINC (Logical Observation Identifiers Names and Codes) are used for results of laboratory tests. ICD (International Classification of Diseases) is used to code for diagnoses. Standardized formats are necessary to ensure interoperability and the ability to transmit and receive data.

27. B: The area of informatics that is most invested in assisting patients to utilized health-enabling technologies to prevent, monitor, and manage disease is consumer health informatics. Guiding patients toward self-management is an important goal of consumer health informatics, and this can include use of monitoring equipment (blood glucose monitors, cardiac monitors, BP monitors) as well as access to internet resources, such as dieting assistance (LoseIt.com) and sources that allow web-based tracking of important data, such as vital signs.

28) A: According to research, from the clinical nurse's perspective, NANDA-I (North American Nursing Diagnosis Association International) is generally found to be most useful for planning care of patients. NANDA-I is a terminology that allows nurses to identify and classify patient problems in terms of nursing diagnoses. Utilizing this information to generate appropriate interventions and to ensure appropriate outcomes are other uses, although retrieving information is found to be less useful because many EHRs do not allow this type of information retrieval.

29. D: The business concept of "planned obsolescence" is utilized in the field of technology primarily to ensure market demand for products continues. Thus, after a period of time (usually a few years), products may be sunsetted, or phased out, so that they are no longer supported by the vendor. Because of this, healthcare organizations are almost constantly in a planning phase for acquiring new technology—hardware and/or software—in order to maintain functionality.

30. C: Workflow design requires input primarily from clinicians and nurses because these professionals have the best understanding of the processes involved in patient care. IT personnel can carry out the mechanical aspects of creating and coding a workflow design, but may have little knowledge of actual clinical processes. Vendor engineers may understand the process of creating a workflow design and the system capabilities as well, but they lack the experience in the organization to know what design elements are specific to the needs of the organization or staff.

31) A: The best method to assess if staff members lack necessary technological skills is to conduct a gap analysis, which evaluates current performance with target performance and determines the steps needed to move from the current performance level to the target. Gap analysis includes assessing the current situation and identifying current outcomes as well as target outcomes and then outlining processes that will help achieve the desired outcomes. Gaps in performance are identified as well as the resources required to close the gaps.

32. C: In a relational database, "redundancy" refers to duplication of attribute data. Redundancy can cause data to be corrupted or for anomalies to occur. Redundancy is present if the same field (attribute) occurs in more than one table (entity). If an attribute depends on another non-key attribute, it is likely redundant. The process by which redundancy is eliminated is normalization. There are different levels of normalization—first normal form (1NF), second normal form (2NF), and third normal form (3NF).

33. B: The structure of data supported by a hierarchical database is one to many (tree or parent-child) but not many to one because data connects only in descending order. Hierarchical databases are used for simple structures, such as telephone number listings, but are not adequate for the current demands of information storage; so hierarchical databases have generally been replaced with relational databases, which are built on a table structure and allow both one-to-many and many-to-one relationships.

34. D: The primary disadvantage to an alert that requires manual activation for viewing is that the healthcare providers may not activate the alert unless failing to do so results in a hard stop. However, if the information is critical or should be read in all circumstances, then the alert should be automated to save the user the extra step of activating the alarm. Alerts should be carefully designed so that they are meaningful because excessive alerts tend to be ignored or overridden.

35. C: When utilizing SAS Enterprise guide to query a database, if the derived data are to be saved permanently, the correct format is the data table. The data are saved and not updated until a query is rerun to gain additional information. With the data view format, the data are continually updated

- 176 -

each time the results are opened and historical data are not saved. The report format is especially formatted so that it can be presented with options including HTML, PDF, text, or RTF but tasks cannot be completed for results in this format.

36. A: When a device (such as an input or output device) is attached to an operating system, the device is undefined if the system is not able to recognize the device. Other possible states include defined (device information is in the database but not available to the system), available (device information is in the database and configured to the operating system), and unavailable (device information is present in its driver but the device is not available).

37. D: A configuration report contains data about the system, hardware, software, workstations, and servers. Because system information is stored in various areas, a utility is utilized to automatically generate a configuration report. An informational report includes data derived from databases. An error/exception report is issued for faults or abnormal data results. A baseline report (usually generated automatically) shows how the system or parts of the system compare to a pre-established baseline.

38. B: The ethical principle that is most represented in the AMIA Code of Ethics (*Principles of professional and ethical conduct for AMIA members*) is beneficence, which focuses on fidelity and preventing harm to others and carrying out actions for the benefit of others. Beneficence is represented in about 65% of the guidelines. The code includes ethical guidelines for interactions with patients (including guardians and authorized representatives), and with colleagues, institutions, and society and research.

39. A: During the phase of technical development, a constructive assessment of the cognitive aspects could evaluate the response to the effort needed to document in the EHR while interviewing a patient because the user's attention must be focused in two different areas—the patient and the computer terminal. Ergonomic aspects include direct dialog with the system; the number of screens that must be accessed in order to carry out an activity, such as with transferring a patient, or the number of mouse clicks needed.

40. C: When conducting technical verifications to determine if a system should become operational, the most difficult assessment is usually of interoperability, especially with how different systems function together, such as the EHR and the radiology information system. Testing should evaluate how quickly, efficiently, and accurately data can be transmitted and how the system responds to changes, such as cancellation of an order or a change in patient's condition or location (such as a transfer from a medical-surgical unit to critical care).

41. D: If during observational testing for the adaptation phase of an information system, the informatics nurse observes users taking notes of data to enter into the system later when they have more time, this suggests an ergonomic problem in dialoging with the system and requires further assessment to determine if the user interface is not adequately intuitive, if too many screen actions (scrolling, clicking) are required, or if the system responds too slowly.

42. C: The purpose of a functionality assessment of an information system is to determine if the system complies with the work processes and if it supports the workflow of the users. If, for example, the system is unable to adequately handle a particular kind of data, this may jeopardize the entire system. Testing for functionality may include validating software through third parties as well as conducting integration tests and non-regression tests. All different functions should be tested.

43. A: During the explorative phase of selecting an information system, the assessment method that is most useful in order to observe the practices in an organization and to identify those agents controlling change is a field study, which obtains data from the work environment itself. Data may be obtained by direct observation as well as one-on-one interviews, questionnaires, and surveys. Those conducting the field study may do so as a complete observer (not interacting) or as a participant.

44. B: According to the HL7 group, the three different types of interoperability are:
- Technical: Systems are able to connect with one other and exchange data without error.
- Semantic: Data is shared among the different systems and interpreted and understood in the exact same manner in each system.
- Process/Social: The system is able to integrate into the workflow and promote the quality of care by providing usability through carefully-designed interfaces and allowing users to access and input information efficiently.

45. D: The National Drug Code (NDC) used for barcoding of medications is recommended by the FDA for use on all inpatient medications and vaccines, applied at the unit dose to decrease the risks of medication errors. The NDC comprises a code of 10 or 11 digits divided into 3 sections:
- Labeler code (4 to 5 digits): Assigned by the FDA and represents the manufacturer, re-packager, or distributer.
- Product code (3 to 4 digits): Assigned by the labeler and describes the medication, strength, and dose.
- Package code (1 to 2 digits): Assigned by the labeler and describes the package form and size.

46. A: HL7 CDA (Clinical Document Architecture) is a standard utilized for document exchange and is appropriate for any clinical document that might contain a signature, such as the discharge summary, prescriptions, and history and physical examination. HL7 CDA utilizes XML language, which allows for documents to be read by human beings (textual) or processed electronically (structured). However, use of HL7 CDA is not currently mandated in the United States, so its use is limited but expected to expand.

47. C: A primary advantage of coded data over free text is that coded data ensure consistent/standardized vocabulary. The coded entries allow improved capture for data mining with no loss of data, such as may occur with illegible or incomplete narrative documentation or lost paper documents. However, the limitations of the vocabulary may result in a less complete picture than free text narrative documentation. While systems generally allow the option of free text, this information is not coded, so this may affect data analysis.

48. D: The agency/organization that develops standards for information systems to support documentation of nursing practice is the ANA (American Nurses Association) through its Nursing Information and Data Set Evaluation Center (NIDSEC). The ANA also evaluates information systems that are voluntarily submitted to the organization to determine if they meet the standards. The ANA Committee on Nursing Practice Information Infrastructure (CNPII) reviews and recognizes taxonomies, nomenclatures, and vocabularies.

49. C: If, when assessing compliance for the EHR with CPOE CDS system, the informatics nurse notes that alerts are frequent and disruptive, resulting in hard stops, and they are routinely

overridden or ignored, the best solution is probably to implement tiered alerts. With tiered alerts, critical alerts (such as for drug-drug interaction) would be displayed automatically and would require action to proceed (hard stop) and disallow overrides, while other alerts may be presented automatically but still allow overrides. A third category of alerts may require no action or overrides.

50. B: NMMDS (Nursing Management Minimum Data Set) is a data element set utilized for nursing administration. NMMDS comprises three categories: (1) nursing care (diagnosis, intervention, outcomes, intensity of care), (2) patient/client demographics (ID, birthdate, gender, race, ethnicity, residence), and (3) service elements (unique numbers for facility/service agency and patient, number of nurse healthcare providers, encounter data, discharge/termination date, patient disposition, and expected payer).

51. A: The CDS intervention that targets preventive care is a recommendation for immunization. Immunization recommendations may target all patients or specific types of patients. CDS may also provide a list of possible diagnoses associated with patient symptoms, reminders of drug interactions, alerts that a prescribed medication is not in the formulary (a cost reduction intervention), planning guides (such as treatment guidelines and drug alerts), and care plans and order sets (to improve efficiency).

52. C: If the CDS system recommends a therapy that the clinician ignores, the system generally takes no further action, as the CDS system only makes recommendations based on inputted data, but the clinician makes the final determination as to whether to follow the recommendation or not. CDS systems are comprised of a base of knowledge, a program that utilizes this knowledge base in assessing patient-specific information, and a method of communicating the recommendations, such as through alerts.

53. D: In terms of information, "longevity" refers to information being usable beyond the current clinical situation so that it has extended usefulness. Accessibility refers to information being easily accessible in order to provide quality care. Ubiquity refers to the need to be able to access information at any location and at any time. Reusability refers to the ability to utilize information for a variety of different purposes, such as for clinical care and data mining.

54. B: According to the International Technical Standard ISO 18104:2003, for a nursing action to be valid it must include at least action and target. For example, a nursing action such as checking blood pressure includes an action (checking) and a target (blood pressure). The standard also lays out the requirements for a nursing diagnosis, which must include both a focus and a judgment. For example, "risk for" (judgment) "seizures" (focus).

55. A: If developing a chart to display data about the age distribution of patients admitted to the oncology department, a useful type of graphic display is a scattergram, which has an X (age) and Y (admissions) axis in order to show the relationship between two variables (in this case admissions to the unit by date and age). A data point is applied for each admission, corresponding to the patient's age. Once the data are charted, then the data are reviewed to determine if a pattern has emerged.

56. B: Considering ethical implications for data dissemination, data that contain ID codes that are linked to names, which are not divulged, would be classified as potentially identifiable because a data user could ostensibly obtain a list of codes and names to identify individuals. Anonymous data contain no identifying information whatsoever because none was collected. Identifiable data

contain names and/or other identifying information. De-identified data has had identifying information removed.

57. D: The governmental agency responsible for oversight of HIPAA's Privacy Rule is the Office of Civil Rights (OCR), which is part of the Department of Health and Human Services (DHHS). An organization must have procedures in place to limit access to PHI and to limit disclosures to only authorized personnel. HIPAA's Privacy Rule protects data in the EHR as well as personal communications between the patient and healthcare providers. Billing information is also protected.

58. A: When integrating data analysis into the performance improvement process, the model of integration that includes developing multidisciplinary teams that function in different areas but all report to the same project manager is organizational because the focus is on not only improving processes at the departmental level but also on achieving work toward a common organizational goal. The project manager may work with team leaders to identify and prioritize projects but is ultimately responsible for ensuring that organizational goals are met.

59. B: High fidelity simulation involves use of actual target equipment such as computers and test software, as part of training so that the users have a realistic training experience. High fidelity simulations usually provide the best learning experience but are the most expensive because of equipment costs. To reduce costs, the test software may be placed on computers that also use a live version of the software and are utilized for patient care. However, the test software and user interface must be easily identifiable and distinguishable from the live version.

60. D: The type of component suitability testing that determines whether or not an input produces the correct output by using test cases is black box testing, which is a form of functional testing. The test cases should focus on the profile of the operating system (specifications/requirement) and should include activation of as many codes as possible so that faults are not missed. Testers need to understand what the software should do but do not need to understand how the software carries out its functions. Black box testing includes decision table testing, all-pairs testing, and boundary value analysis.

61. B: The technical standard that applies to accessibility of software is ISO 9241-171:2008. The International Organization of Standardization (ISO) is a non-governmental network of institutes that develop and publish voluntary standards that are used internationally in a wide variety of fields. The ISO 9241 series relate to accessibility with ISO 9241-20:2009 providing standards for information/communication technology (equipment and services) and ISO 9241-151:2008 provides standards for World Wide Web user interfaces. ISO 900:2008 provides standards for quality management systems and ISO 639-4:2010 for information security management.

62. C: VoIP (Voice over Internet Protocol) encodes audio files into digital files so that they can be streamed over the internet. VoIP is utilized for internet telephone services, such as Vonage. VoIP also allows multimedia transmission, FAX transmission, and text messaging (SMS—short messaging service). VoIP technology is available on many smartphones and computers. Some systems that utilize VoIP are closed to subscribers only (such as Skype) while others are open (such as Google Talk).

63. B: For archiving data, both federal and state regulations (which sometimes require longer storage than federal regulations) may apply, and they may be different. Federal regulations per the HIPAA Privacy Rule require that clinical health records of living adults be maintained securely for

at least 6 years, although records must be maintained for only 2 years after a patient's death. Records of infants born in a healthcare facility must be maintained until the child is 18 years old. The FDA requires that mammography records be stored for 10 years or until the time another mammogram is taken.

64. A: A primary advantage of tiered archival storage is cost effectiveness. With tiered storage, different storage devices are used for different data with data most important to an organization stored on faster equipment and older or less important data stored on slower and less expensive equipment. Software programs are used to automate movement of data from one tier to another or to remove data, such as when federal or state regulations no longer require storage of the data.

65. C: The domain suffix likely to deliver the most reliable information is *.gov*, such as cms.gov and HHS.gov. Because there are many kinds of organizations, the suffix *.org* may or not yield reliable information. Major healthcare organizations, such as the American Heart Association (heart.org), are usually reliable. The suffix *.com* is used for all different types of webpages so there is little expectation of reliability. The suffix *.edu* indicates an educational institution, but in many cases all staff members and all students may have information on sites using the *.edu* suffix with varying degrees of reliability.

66. D: The goal of translational research is to translate medical/nursing research into interventions, so that it is a basis for evidence-based practice. An important factor in translational research is that the scientific aspects of the research are understood by the healthcare providers so that they comply with the recommended interventions. One problem associated with translating research into interventions is that research often presents the most positive aspects of change rather than the negative, so problems may arise during application.

67. A: In an evidence hierarchy, the type of evidence that would have the highest priority is meta-analysis, which involves analysis of multiple research projects dealing with the same or similar problem. The hierarchy continues with individual experimental studies, quasi-experimental studies, non-experimental studies, program evaluations, and expert opinion. Interestingly, expert opinion is the least valid type of evidence because it is based on subjective analysis rather than objective, even though expert opinion is often highly valued.

68. D: When planning staff training for EHR implementation, the informatics nurse should keep in mind that the best retention is likely to occur if the participants practice using the EHR with real equipment, which includes both speaking (providing feedback, asking questions) and doing. Retention at 24 hours is about 90% with this method of instruction. The least effective method of retention is reading, which results in only about 10% comprehension, followed by listening (20%), viewing (30%), listening and viewing (50%), and speaking and writing (70%).

69. A: Considering the systems in a healthcare organization, a suprasystem includes not only the subsystems, such as nursing and radiology, but also external elements that affect the organization, such as accrediting agencies and the public health department, as well as the sociopolitical environment. An open system allows exchanges between subsystems (such as between the laboratory and nursing) while a closed system is completely contained and does not interact with other systems; closed systems rarely occur nowadays.

70. C: If the informatics nurse wants to make training materials available in audio and video format for staff members, the best method is probably to provide downloadable digital materials that can be loaded onto mobile devices, such as smartphones, iPods, tablets, PDAs, and netbooks, because

these mobile devices are in common use. Videos and audio presentations (such as podcasts) should usually be limited to about 10 minutes per lesson because people tend to lose concentration after 10 to 15 minutes.

71. B: If a hospital develops a social media site to provide informational content to consumers but finds that it has almost no traffic, the best solution is to conduct surveys to determine what consumers want and what they like or dislike about the site and then re-evaluate. Reasons for lack of traffic may include poor design, poor marketing, and/or inadequate content. Branding is an important consideration and formatting should be consistent with the same logo, fonts, and colors utilized for all content.

72. C: If, as project manager, the informatics nurse has encountered a team member who talks compulsively during meetings and ignores suggestions that all team members participate, the best solution is to discuss the problem face-to-face outside of the meeting in a non-confrontational manner, stressing the need to hear from all team members while expressing value for the team member's participation. Assigning a specific task or role may help, such as taking minutes, and may focus the person's attention away from the need to talk constantly.

73. A: When sending a reminder of a team meeting by E-mail, the most important information to include in the E-mail is the purpose (problem solving, brainstorming, disseminating information) and the agenda. The team leader should develop the agenda that outlines the categories (information, implementation, development, change) of each agenda item prior to scheduling the meeting if possible or long enough in advance that team members have time to consider the agenda and gather any necessary information or materials.

74. A: If the information programmed in a CDS system is incorrect and a patient suffers harm because of this, the person responsible for the incorrect information may be accused of negligent misstatement because this form of negligence does not require a contractual agreement or duty to care. The "experts," in this case are the person who provided the information, and who has a responsibility to ensure that information is correct, and the programmer who ensures that the information is correctly inputted.

75. D: According to Ruesch, the five major elements that are required for communication are (1) sender, (2) message (includes not only words stated or written but also nonverbal communications), (3) receiver, (4) feedback (the response to the message), and (5) context (setting, mood, relationship between sender and receiver). The three major operations associated with communication include (1) perception, (2) evaluation, and (3) transmission.

76. B: With Total Quality Management (TQM), the primary focus is on satisfying the needs of the customers. The organization conducts various assessments (surveys, interviews, focus groups) to determine customer needs and engages the entire organization at all levels in the improvement process with teamwork and participation encouraged. Measurement is central to TQM's processes, so criteria are identified through brainstorming and other methods, and quality improvement is measured. For TQM to be successful, it must be supported by top management.

77. A: The Quality and Safety Education for Nurses (QSEN) project's informatics competency ("Use information and technology to communicate, manage knowledge, mitigate error, and support decision making") includes the 3 elements of KSAs:

- Knowledge: Ability to evaluate benefits and strengths and weaknesses, evaluate communication technologies, determine information essential to a patient care database, and demonstrate understanding of taxonomy and terminology.
- Skills: Participation, selection, implementation, promotion, and evaluation.
- Attitude: Values information/communication technologies, need for consensus and collaboration, and use of standardized terminologies.

78. C: When carrying out an SQL query of a relational database, BETWEEN is classified as a *logical* operator. Logical operators are words, while arithmetic and comparison operators are symbols. Operators are used primarily in WHERE clauses when carrying out operations, such as making comparisons.
- Logical: ALL, AND, ANY, BETWEEN, EXISTS, IN, LIKE, NOT (negate operator), OR, IS NULL, and UNIQUE.
- Arithmetic: +, -, *, /, %.
- Comparison: =, !=, <>, >, <, >=, <=, !<, !>.

79. B: While all of these are important issues, if the informatics nurse has found a new application that may enhance the existing EHR with CPOE CDS system, the first concern before recommending the application is compatibility. If the application will not work within the existing system or it requires extensive workaround, then it is not a good choice. The informatics nurse should consult with the vendor as well as IT personnel and programmers to determine whether there are compatibility issues.

80. D: An example of "web surfing" is navigating the internet by clicking links for one site after another. Web surfing may be intentional in the sense that the person is searching for a specific type of information, but this is a relatively ineffective way of gathering information. Most often, web surfing is recreational and the person is randomly clicking on various links, such as may occur when a person is clicking links in the newsfeed on Facebook.

81. B: With encryption of data, "stickiness" refers to the degree to which encryption persists when encrypted data are moved from one site to another, such as from one disk to another. Many types of encryption are only valid when the data are "at rest" or stored in one location or within one network. For example, a file that is encrypted in a network may lose encryption if it is sent as an E-mail attachment, so the stickiness of encryption is an important consideration when data must be transmitted outside the system.

82. A: When decommissioning a computer information system (CIS), one of the purposes of the Records Management Plan (RMP) is to ensure disposition of data corresponds to federal/state regulations so that data that must be retained is properly archived and other data disposed of correctly. All stored data must be evaluated and disposition determined and outlined in a plan that includes policies and procedures. Intellectual property rights should be evaluated to determine if these rights will affect disposition of data.

83. D: A one-on-one interview is an example of a qualitative approach to obtaining user feedback about a computer information system. Qualitative data are narrative rather than numerical (quantitative) although some quantitative approaches may be applied to qualitative data. Qualitative feedback is utilized to determine the users' perceptions of the information system and to help provide cause. For example, if quantitative data show increased documentation errors, qualitative research may be able to help ascertain the reason.

84. C: The three-phase change management process (Prosci) includes:
- Phase I, preparing for change: Define the strategy for managing change and organize and prepare the change management team.
- Phase II, managing change: Develop plans for change management and begin the process of change by implementing plans.
- Phase III: reinforcing change: Identify and manage resistance and gaps and obtain and evaluate feedback, taking whatever steps are necessary to correct problems and ensure positive outcomes.

85. C: Process mapping may be done at 3 different levels:
- Macro level: A general overview of a process with many component parts, such as admission procedures.
- Mini level: Process steps in a procedure that involves a number of different tasks, such as completing wound assessment, irrigation, and dressing change or transferring a patient.
- Micro level: Process steps in detail that one individual will take to carry out one procedure, such as completing a blood draw.

86. A: A chart migration plan should be formulated before going live with an EHR to ensure that important patient data are not lost or are unavailable. The migration plan should outline the steps to transferring data from paper charts to the EHR, including the timeframe, who is responsible, and what data are to be transferred. Because of the changing nature of patients' conditions and census, much data must be transferred in a short period of time and this can pose numerous logistical problems.

87. B: The GUI (graphical user interface) facilitates interaction between the user and the computer. The GUI provides a means of navigating within the computer environment. The GUI is part of the computer operating system. It is the "desktop" screen, usually with icons that can be activated by clicking them with a mouse or selecting with a trackball or other device. The design of the GUI should be intuitive so that the user can determine what actions to take without written instructions.

88. D: The primary disadvantage to scanning paper documents into an EHR rather than coding them is that the data cannot be mined. If only a few patient records are involved, the problem may not be of statistical concern, but in a large institution with large numbers of patients, this may skew data. During implementation of an EHR, the organization should determine what information is most critical and that information should be coded even if the documents are scanned. The same type of problem arises if staff uses excessive free text in documentation.

89. A: As part of the American Recovery and Reinvestment Act (ARRA), the Office of the National Coordinator for Health Information Technology (ONC) established 62 Regional Extension Centers (RECs) in order to assist healthcare organizations to adopt EHRs. The REC assists healthcare providers to enroll in the REC program, implement an EHR, and achieve stage 1 of meaningful use. The REC assists in health IT training, selection of vendors, workflow redesign, privacy and security issues, and technical issues.

90. D: When notified that a costly upgrade to the EHR is scheduled for implementation within the next few months, the first step should be to request details and a demonstration. Most vendors will provide a demo version so that the organization can have a clear idea of the changes. Updates, such as adding new medications to the medication list, are frequent and usually involve no disruption in

workflow or utilization of the EHR, but upgrades may be more problematic so they must be thoroughly assessed. Upgrades often improve functioning or respond to changes in regulations or technology.

91. C: When the informatics nurse notes that there has been a marked increase in help-desk tickets to one hospital unit, the first action should be to analyze the types of help-desk tickets to determine if, for example, they relate to the same or similar problems or to various types of problems. Then, the informatics nurse should interview the help desk staff members about the types of problems and their perceptions of the causes. After this, the informatics nurse should interview the staff members on the unit. Additional training may or may not be needed, depending on the results of the investigation.

92. B: An example of aggregate data is hospital census data for the state. Aggregate data is derived from a compilation of data from different sources, so the data that is presented as a separate entity (census data) is derived from multiple more discrete data items, such as census reports from each hospital, city, and county. Other types of aggregate data include financial reports, demographic information, and summary reports. Aggregate data by their nature do not provide detailed information.

93. D: When considering improvements to workflow processes, the first issue to address is whether steps in a process can be eliminated because the goal is to simplify while still maintaining the integrity of the process. Eliminating steps may result from purchasing of new equipment, altering product design, or changing the environment (such as carrying out a process at point of care rather than in another area). In some cases, steps may be simplified by combining some steps with others or by changing the order of steps.

94. A: If the hospital is considering a telemedicine venture that would provide internet consultation and treatment to rural patients in four states, the first concern is licensure. There is no national licensure or consensus about licensure for interstate treatment and prescription, so each state must be queried to determine the requirements for telemedicine. In some cases, physicians must be licensed in each state. Some states allow a specified number of consultations without state licensure. Some states have a special telemedicine license.

95. C: Considering cloud architecture, if software applications are hosted by the vendor and then distributed to the organization via the internet, this model is referred to as software as a service (SAS). (The SAS designation can be confusing because it can also refer to storage or security as a service.) With infrastructure as a service, the vendor hosts not only the software applications but also hardware, servers, and storage. With platform as a service, the vendor provides hardware and software tools needed for running or developing applications.

96. D: If an institution permits personalized order sets for the CPOE CDS system because of a specialized treatment center, the order sets should be reviewed at least annually. While personalized order sets are not recommended, they are permitted but should be developed following guidelines from the Institute for Safe Medication Practices (ISMP) and should include dose, dose form, route, and frequency. The 10 order sets that are available (including chest pain management, insulin administration, OB administration) are based on best evidence practices.

97. B: In an EHR, orderable items, such as radiology tests and medications, should be requested by browsing through an alphabetical listing. Queries and key word searches using free text should not be necessary. For medications, the listings should include both generic names and brand names,

and various word orders should be used for treatments, such as "ultrasound, bladder" or "bladder ultrasound." Users should be able to simply click on the item of choice to generate an order.

98. D: If laboratory results input into the EHR show critical values, the clinician should be notified verbally immediately to ensure that the clinician has received the information, and the notification should be documented. The notification may be per telephone or face-to-face communication, but text messages are not sufficient, even if the clinician responds to the message, because the sender cannot legally verify that the actual receiver of the message was the clinician.

99. A: A collection of data about one particular hospital unit or a specific topic to facilitate decision-making by administration is a data mart. This may be as small as one database or may be a compilation of databases, but is generally a subset of a data warehouse (AKA enterprise data warehouse), which is a very large database or storage depository with integrated data. The data warehouse includes all of an organization's databases. The data warehouse may be utilized for reporting of data as well as data mining for analysis.

100. C: As a project manager who is charged with creating a number of teams to facilitate transition to an EHR, the informatics nurse should limit team size to fewer than 10 people because larger teams often lose focus and have competing interests. Team members should have complementary skills and should be interdisciplinary, representing the various interests. Teams should have some degree of autonomy and flexibility even though working on a specific mandate.

101. D: The effective display of patient data for clinical decision-making requires that information be rapidly available with minimal cognitive effort. Multiple displays on one screen are distracting and slow cognitive processing of data. The decision tree is a common presentation with potential options, consequences, and expected outcomes. Other types of presentations include tables, various types of graphs, and icons. In most cases, multiple modes of presentation of data provide the best information. Visual indicators, such as colors, may be used to highlight information, such as abnormal lab results, and pictorial displays can be effective.

102. A: Throughput. The 5 elements in a system include:
- Input: This is what goes into a system in terms of energy or materials.
- Throughput: These are the actions that take place in order to transform input.
- Output: This is the result of the interrelationship between input and processes.
- Evaluation: Monitoring success or failure.
- Feedback: This is information that results from the process and can be used to evaluate the end result.

Bertalanffy believed that all of the elements of a system interact in order to achieve goals, and change in any one element will impact the other elements and alter outcomes.

103. B: Untethered PHRs are standalone and not connected to a particular system or EHR. Information may be carried on a smart card, flash card, CD, or DVD. These pose more security risks than tethered PHRs and require more input from the individual to maintain accurate records. In tethered PHRs, data are tied to a particular system and EHR and often web-based. A secure patient portal is provided so the individual can access all or parts of the records. In networked PHRs, data are derived from multiple sources in a network rather than one system. This allows for more flexibility. In paper/personal files, patient-maintained paper records are contained.

104. D: Aggregate data includes pharmacy transactions, required reports, demographic information, financial information, hazard and safety practices, and most things not included in the clinical record. Medical/clinical data includes patient-specific information regarding the patient, diagnosis, treatment, laboratory findings, consultations, care plans, physician orders, and information related to informed consent and advance directives. The medical record should include records of all procedures, discharge summary, and emergency care records. Knowledge based data includes methods to ensure that staff is provided training, support, research, library services, or other access to information, and good practice guidelines. Comparison data includes internal comparisons or external comparisons to benchmarks or best-practice guidelines.

105. C: Language elements of SQL include:
- Queries: The most commonly used SQL operation, require a SELECT statement.
- Clauses: From, where, group by, having, and order by.
- Expressions: Produce scales and tables.
- Predicates: 3-valued logic (null, true, false) and Boolean truth values.
- Statements: Includes the semicolon (to terminate a statement).

Structured query language (SQL) is a fourth-generation programming language (4GL) that differs from 3GLs, such as Java, in that SQL uses syntax similar to human language to access, manipulate, and retrieve data from relational database management system (RDBMS), which stores data in tables.

106. A: Legitimate infringement is the consideration for greater good of society in regard to individual's right to privacy. Part I, the introduction, of the IMIA Code of Ethics includes the six primary ethical principles: autonomy, equality and justice, beneficence, non-malfeasance, impossibility, and integrity. General principles in the introduction include:
- The right to privacy regarding sharing of personal information and control of types of collection, methods of collection, and storage.
- Open process of data collection with patient informed.
- Security of all data collection and protection from data manipulation.
- Right to access of personal data.
- Infringement of right to privacy with minimum interference.
- Accountability for infringement.

107. B: Change theory:
1. Motivation to change (unfreezing): Dissatisfaction occurs when goals are not met. Previous beliefs are brought into question and survival anxiety occurs. Sometimes learning anxiety about having to learn different strategies causes resistance that can lead to denial, blaming others, and trying to maneuver or bargain without real change.
2. Desire to change (unfrozen): Dissatisfaction is strong enough to override defensive actions and desire to change is strong but these must be coupled with identification of needed changes.
3. Development of permanent change (refreezing): New behavior becomes habitual, often requiring a change in perceptions of self and establishment of new relationships.

108. D: Determining measures of equivalency. Steps to conducting usability studies include:
1. Defining purpose.
2. Evaluating constraints such as time, staff, and resources.

3. Refining components based on evaluation of human-computer interaction (HCI) framework, determining each component and to whom or what it applies, including choosing the most appropriate staff, determining the most important step in a process, determining measures of equivalency, and choosing the setting.
4. Determining emphasis, which may focus on one or more aspects.
5. Selecting methods, which must match purpose and take account of constraints and HCI.

109. A: A cost-benefit analysis uses average cost of an event and the cost of intervention to demonstrate savings. A cost-effective analysis measures the effectiveness of an intervention rather than the monetary savings. Efficacy studies may compare a series of cost-benefit analyses to determine the intervention with the best cost-benefit. They may also be used for process or product evaluation. Cost-utility analysis (CUA) is essentially a subtype of cost-effective analysis, but it is more complex and the results are more difficult to quantify and use to justify expense because cost-utility analysis measures benefit to society in general, such as decreasing teen pregnancy.

110. C: The Unicode Standard coding scheme, used with the Universal Character Set (UCS), is a standardized coding system that has a larger capacity and can be used to represent text for most languages, including Asian. Coding is available to represent technical characters, punctuation, and mathematic symbols. Unicode provides a specific numeric value for each character and can be used across multiple platforms. Unicode comprises approximately 110,000 characters representing all alphabets in the world languages, ideographic sets, and symbols, as well as 100 scripts, and is particularly valuable for making coding accessible internationally. Unicode is utilized in many technologies and operating systems.

111. B: Unauthorized access: Providers sometimes share or expose their passwords to other health care professionals when logging in, allowing others to access information about patients. Other types of misuse include:
- Identity theft: Health records often contain identifying information, such as Social Security numbers and credit card numbers as well as birthdates and addresses.
- Privacy violations: Even those authorized to access a patient's record may share private information with others, such as family or friends.
- Security breach: Data is vulnerable to security breach because of careless or inadequate security, especially when various business associates, such as billing companies, have access to private information.

112. A: The primary purpose of sending an RFI to a variety of vendors is to help in the elimination and selection process. Topics for questions may include:
- History and financial status of company.
- Lists of current users of company's product and numbers of sites.
- Information about system architecture.
- Hardware/software requirements.
- User support.
- Equipment support/maintenance.
- Ability of equipment to integrate with other systems.

Requests for information (RFI) are used early in system analysis to gather information from various vendors, often in conjunction with requests for proposal (RFP) and requests for quote (RFQ).

113. D: Bloom's taxonomy describes 3 types of learning:

- Cognitive: Learning and gaining intellectual skills and mastering categories of effective learning (knowledge, comprehension, application, analysis, synthesis, and evaluation).
- Affective: Recognizing categories of feelings and values from simple to complex (receiving and responding to phenomena, valuing, organizing and internalizing values).
- Psychomotor: Mastering motor skills necessary for independence, following a progression from simple to complex (perception, set, guided response, mechanism, complex overt response, adaptation, origination).

114. C: Wound AND povidone-iodine NOT antibiotics. Boolean searching is often used with truncations and wildcards:
- Truncations: "Finan*" provides all words that begin with those letters, such as "finance," "financial," and "financed."
- Wildcards: "m?n" or "m*n" provides "man" and "men."
- AND: "Wound AND antibiotic" produces all documents that contain both words.
- OR: "Wound OR Infect* OR ulcer" produces documents that contain "wound" and either "infect*" or "ulcer." This query is especially useful to search for a number of synonyms or variant spellings.
- NOT: Wound AND povidone-iodine NOT antibiotic NOT antimicrobial. NOT is used to exclude keywords.

115. B: The first step to knowledge discovery in databases (KDD) is data selection. Other steps include pre-processing (assembling target data set and cleaning data of noise), transforming data, data mining, and interpreting of results. KDD is a method to identify patterns and relationships in large amounts of data, such as the identification of risk factors or effectiveness of interventions. KDD may utilize data perturbation, the hiding of confidential information (such as name) while maintaining the basic information in the database, and data mining.

116. A: According to the privacy rule, protected information includes any information included in the medical record, conversations between the doctor and other health care providers, billing information, and any other forms of health information. According to the security rule, any electronic health information must be secure and protected against threats, hazards, or nonpermitted disclosures. Implementation specifications must be addressed for any adopted standards. Security requirements include limiting access to those authorized, use of unique identifiers for each user, automatic logoff, encryption and decryption of protected health care information, authentication that health care data have not been altered/destroyed, monitoring of logins, authentication, and security of transmission.

117. B: Gap analysis is used to determine the steps required to move from a current state or actual performance or situation to a new one or potential performance or situation, and the "gap" between the two that requires action or resources. Steps to gap analysis include:
- Assessing the current situation and listing important factors, such as performance levels, costs, staffing, and satisfaction, and all processes.
- Identifying the current outcomes of processes.
- Identifying the target outcomes for projected processes.
- Outlining the process required to achieve target outcomes.
- Identifying the gaps that are present.
- Identifying resources and methods to close the gaps.

118. D: Data mining is the analysis (often automatic) of large amounts of data to identify underlying or hidden patterns. The steps to data mining include detecting anomalies, identifying relationships, clustering, classifying, regressing, and summarizing. The effectiveness of data mining depends on many factors, such as hardware and software applications. Data mining may identify similar groupings in data, and these groups can then be further analyzed. Data mining may be applied to multiple patients' electronic health records to generate information about the need for further examination or interventions.

119. B: Switching to Voice–over-Internet Protocol (VoIP) devices and eliminating landline telephones is a cost-saving measure because voice and data can use the same network. VoIP includes the protocols and technology involved in allowing audio and multimedia transmission, such as audio, FAX, messaging, and short message service (SMS), which is text messaging, over the internet. VoIP is also referred to as broadband telephone or internet telephone, and companies such as Vonage market their service as an alternative to landline telephones. VoIP allows SMS or calls from nonphone devices with access to Wi-Fi, 3G, or 4G.

120. A: Orem's general theory of nursing is based on 3 theories: self-care, self-care deficit, and nursing systems. Neuman's total-person systems model focuses on how the individual reacts to stress through mechanisms of defense and resistance and how this feedback affects that individual's stability. Interventions include primary, secondary, and tertiary. Orlando's nursing process theory includes the behavior of the patient, the nurse's reaction, and the subsequent nurse actions. Huff's crisis theory considers those stress-related events that are turning points in a person's life and can lead to danger or to opportunity.

121. C: HL7 is the messaging standard used to communicate clinical data and is utilized by virtually all medical informatics systems to promote interoperability and the exchange of information. ASTM provides standards for a wide range of health care elements, including equipment, storage, and communication. ASTM has also developed security standards for the field of health care informatics. IEEE provides standards for communication networks, including standards for the utilization of point-of-care instruments. DICOM provides standards utilized in transmitting medical images, such as radiographs.

122. A: A hub serves as a connecting device and brings network data together. For example, a typical configuration is a hub connecting workstations, printers, and a server. A bridge connects networks at the data link level. A router determines data's destination. Another communication device is a gateway, which is utilized to connect different networks operating under different protocols. A switch, which may comprise a router or a gateway, sends data to the correct destination.

123. D: The American Recovery and Reinvestment Act of 2009 (ARRA) included the Health Information Technology for Economic and Clinical Health (HITECH) Act. Security provisions include the following:
- Individuals and HHS must be notified of breach in security of personal health information.
- Business partners must meet security regulations or face penalties.
- The sale/marketing of personal health information is restricted.
- Individuals must have access to electronic health information.
- Individuals must be informed of disclosures of personal health information.

HITECH provides incentive payments to Medicare practitioners to adopt EHRs. Additionally, HITECH provides penalties in the form of reduced Medicare payments for those who do not adopt EHRs, unless exempted.

124. C: A PIN is an example of a disconnected token because no additional equipment is required. Smart cards and USB tokens are connected tokens and an RFID device is contactless. Tokens are items used to authenticate a person's identity and allow access to a system. They commonly require the use of not only the token but also a PIN or user name and password. Some devices, such as the SecureID token by RSA generate one-time passwords (OTPs). Tokens may be in the form of access cards, which may utilize different technologies such as photos, optical coding, electric circuits, and magnetic strips.

125. C: Channel capacity determines the amount of information that can be transmitted with the smallest rate of error. Signal-to-noise (S/N) indicates the ratio between a signal's magnitude and interfering "noise" magnitude. Entropy refers to the amount of energy, code or bits, required to communicate or store one symbol in the communication process. The lower the entropy, the more efficient the process of communication. The information theory (Shannon) identified 3 steps in communication: encoding, transmitting, and decoding.

126. A: The Theory of Cognitive Dissonance (Festinger) states that individuals attempt to escape dissonance and avoid inconsistencies between their beliefs and actions. If dissonance occurs, then beliefs and ideas are more likely to change than actions or behavior. To avoid dissonance, people may avoid individuals or situations in which dissonance occurs. When faced with dissonance, the person can:
- Change one cognition (piece of knowledge) to match others or change all to bring them in line.
- Eliminate one cognition or add more to bring about consonance.
- Alter the importance of cognitions.

127. D: Sensitivity: Data should include all positive cases, taking into account variables, decreasing the number of false negatives.
- Specificity: Data should include only those cases specific to the needs of the measurement and exclude those that may be similar but are a different population, decreasing the number of false positives.
- Stratification: Data should be classified according to subsets, taking variables into consideration.
- Validity: Data should measure the target adequately, so that the results have predictive value.
- Recordability: The tool/indicator should collect and measure the necessary data.
- Reliability: Results should be reproducible.
- Usability: The tool or indicator should be easy to utilize and understand.

128. B: A dashboard (also called a digital dashboard), like the dashboard in a car, is an easy to access and read computer program that integrates a variety of performance measures or key indicators into one display (usually with graphs or charts) to provide an overview of an organization. It might include data regarding patient satisfaction, infection rates, financial status, or any other measurement that is important to assess performance. The dashboard provides a running picture of the status of the department or organization at any point in time, and may be updated as desired, such as daily, weekly, or monthly.

129. C: When highlighting text, underlining is more evident than italicizing and bolding because screens have different lighting and resolution. Text against a colored background, especially a deep color, is difficult to read. Colored fonts may be used sparingly to highlight different types of information. Using a variety of fonts and multiple sizes on one screen can be very distracting. Long paragraphs should be avoided and information broken into small chunks with adequate white space to rest the eyes. Font size should be 12 to 14 for standard text with greater size for headings.

130. D: Cognitive walkthrough is one method to assess the users' abilities to understand the model and its purpose, to produce the desired actions, and to determine if users understand which is the right action and whether they understand system feedback. The "think aloud" procedure is used while participants utilize a product and carry out the steps in a process, noting any usability problems, including the ability to learn the process without formal training. Sessions may be audiotaped or videotaped for later evaluation.

131. B: User acceptance testing (UAT) is done to determine the end-user's willingness to utilize computer technology and software in the way in which they are designed, and should begin with analyzing the basic requirements of the system and the organization. Subsequent steps include:
- Identifying the end-user acceptance scenarios.
- Describing a testing plan, including different severity levels based on real-world conditions.
- Designing the testing plan and test cases, considering risks and the skills of the end-users.
- Conducting the tests.
- Evaluating and recording results.

132. A: The primary focus of HCI is usability related to human performance during interactions with computers in different contexts, including concerns regarding overall ease of use, difficulty in learning, efficiency, satisfaction, ability to carry out error-free interactions, and ability of the computer system to match the tasks. Another focus is the mental model of users, the idea that the users have regarding interactions with computers based on knowledge and experience. This mental model should be consistent with the concept or design of the model, so the goal is to find a design that helps promote an effective mental model.

133. C: When a person is sitting and working at a computer, the elbows should be bent at a 90-degree angle and wrists held straight. The seat of the chair should be adjusted so that the person's feet are flat on the floor (or on a foot stool if the person is short) with the knees also bent at a 90-degree angle. The chair should provide support in the lower back, and the angle of the back of the chair to the seat should be 90 degrees.

134. D: Social Exchange Theory describes communication as an exchange system in which people attempt to negotiate a return on their "investment." Social Penetration Theory describes the manner in which people use communication to develop closeness to others, proceeding from superficial communication to more explicit self-disclosure. Communication Accommodation Theory explains why people alter their communication styles. Individuals may practice convergence or divergence. Spiral of Silence Theory looks at the role mass media has in influencing communication and suggests that people fear isolation, so they conform to public opinions as espoused by mass media and mute dissent.

135. B: Gross negligence. Negligence indicates that *proper care* has not been provided, based on established standards. Reasonable care uses rationale for decision-making in relation to providing care. Types of negligence:

- Negligent conduct indicates that an individual failed to provide reasonable care or to protect/assist another, based on standards and expertise.
- Gross negligence is willfully providing inadequate care while disregarding the safety and security of another.
- Contributory negligence involves the injured party contributing to his/her own harm.
- Comparative negligence attempts to determine what percentage amount of negligence is attributed to each individual involved.

136. C: Elements of a PHR should include:
- The PHR discloses who entered data and when as well as who has accessed the data.
- The individual has the ability to control the PHR.
- The information in the PHR is comprehensive and covers the patient's lifetime.
- The information in the PHR derives from all health care providers.
- The PHR can be easily accessible at any time from any location with access.
- The information contained in the PHR is secure and cannot be accessed without proper authorization.
- Exchange of information with different health care providers across the health care system is efficient.

137. A: Those applying for incentive payments must use certified EHR systems that have demonstrated they can store and share patient data securely, maintaining privacy, and that they will begin participation as soon as possible. Incentive payment will not begin until the program is launched. The CMS has established Medicare and Medicaid incentive programs for adoption, upgrade, and/or utilization of electronic health records. CMS conducts the Medicare EHR incentive program and the state's Medicaid EHR incentive programs. Physicians and chiropractors are eligible to participate in the Medicare program, and nurse practitioners, nurse-midwives, dentists, and physician assistants may also qualify to participate in the Medicaid programs.

138. C: Rules applied to trending analysis:
- Astronomical value: Data point unrelated to other points indicates sentinel event or special cause variation.
- Run (shift): ≥ 7 consecutive data points all above or all below the median (run chart) or mean (control chart).
- Trend: ≥ 7 consecutive data points in either ascending or descending order with ≥ 21 total data points or ≥ 6 with fewer than 21 total data points.
- Cycle: Up and down variation forming a sawtooth pattern with 14 successive data points, suggestive of systemic effect on data. If the trend is related to common cause variation, the variation may be demonstrated with 4-11 successive data points.

139. D: Leapfrog Safe Practices Score assesses the progress a health care organization is making on 30 safe practices that Leapfrog has identified as reducing the risk of harm to patients. Leapfrog is a consortium of health care purchasers/employers and has developed a number of initiatives to improve safety. Leapfrog provides an annual Hospital and Quality Safety Survey to assess progress, releases regional data, and encourages voluntary public reporting. Leapfrog has instituted the Leapfrog Hospital Recognition Program (LHRP) as a pay-for-performance program to reward organizations for showing improvement in key measures.

140. B: National Quality Forum's safe practices include managing medications by implementing a computerized prescriber order entry (CPOE) system, using standardizing abbreviations,

maintaining updated medication lists for patients, and including pharmacists in medication management to identify high-alert drugs and dispense drugs in unit doses. Additional safe practices include considering patient's rights and responsibilities, managing information and care, preventing health care–associated infections, providing safe practices for surgery, and providing procedures and ongoing assessment to prevent site-specific or treatment-specific adverse events.

141. C: Devices can be in four different states when connected to a system:
- Undefined: The system does not recognize the device.
- Defined: Information about a specific device is present in the database but not available to the system.
- Available: Information about a device is present in the database and configured to the operating system.
- Not available/Stopped: Information about the device is present in its driver but the device is not available.

142. C: Low-fidelity simulations rely on verbal, print, video, or audio descriptions and often involve discussion of potential actions rather than actual practice. Thus, learners may be presented with a case study or scenario with specific problems and asked to describe the process for dealing with the problems. High-fidelity simulations are those that use real and/or realistic equipment, such as computers, and materials as part of learning. Functional simulations provide practice in one specific area of function. Process simulations utilize mathematics and focus on quantitative analysis.

143. B: Types of system reports that may be available include:
- Error/Exception: Indicate faults or data outside of normal parameters.
- Configuration: Contain data about the system itself, including hardware and software as well as workstations and servers.
- Informational: Often include built-in templates and provide fact-finding to glean information from databases.
- Change: Usually automated and show changes occurring in the system over a period of time.
- Baseline: Usually automated to show how the system or elements of the system compare to a baseline.
- Summary/Management: Show summaries of actions, processes, data.
- Periodic: Issued at predetermined periods, such as monthly claims reports.

144. D: Over-the-shoulder instruction is a learner-centered strategy in which the instructor moves about the classroom monitoring the learner's progress rather than standing at the front of the classroom and lecturing or providing instructor-focused teaching. Most instruction is per computer-assisted instruction (CAI). This strategy allows for one-on-one instruction with individual learners as the instructor sees the need or the learner requests, and the instructor is better able to monitor individual progress. However, many learners may have the same questions, so the instructor may waste time answering the same questions multiple times to individual students.

145. B: When instituting changes, the best approach is to provide honest information about the reasons for changes and how staff will be affected. Resistance to change is common for many people, so coordinating collaborative processes requires anticipating resistance and taking steps to achieve cooperation. Resistance often relates to concerns about job loss, increased responsibilities, and general denial or lack of understanding and frustration. The nurse should be empathetic and patient, allowing people to express their opinions and encouraging their participation.

146. A: In the guided focus teaching model, learning takes place outside of formal classroom with materials provided or recommended by instructor. In an independent study model, the study is geared toward the needs of the individual and can be self-paced. Materials may be web-based or paper-based and may include audio-visual materials. In a cognitive apprenticeship model, Instructors model and learners analyze and apply processes. Cooperative: Small teams work together through a variety of activities to master a subject, with each member responsible for self-learning and the learning of others in the team.

147. D: Typically, the following symbols are used in a process diagram, such as a clinical workflow chart:
- Parallelogram: Input and output (Start/End).
- Arrow: Direction of flow.
- Diamond-shape: Conditional decision (Yes/No or True/False)
- Circle: Connectors with diverging paths with multiple arrows coming in but only one going out.

A variety of other symbols may be used as well to indicate different functions. Flow goes from top to bottom and left to right. Flow charts are particularly useful in helping people to visualize how a process is carried out, to examine a process for problems, and to plan a process.

148. C: Discrete data, usually used to represent the count of something, are those that have a specific value and cannot be further quantified. Because the person creating the database and the person providing data are often different, eliciting the correct discrete data can pose problems, especially if the person providing data is not well versed in database design. One of the first steps to ensuring adequate data is to do a requirement analysis, which can involve eliciting information about data through case studies, interviews, focus groups, and observations.

149. B: CPT codes, developed by the American Medical Association (AMA), define those licensed to provide services and describe medical and surgical treatments, diagnostics, and procedures. The use of CPT codes is mandated by both CMS and HIPAA to provide a uniform language and to aid research. These codes are used primarily for billing purposes for insurances (public and private). HHS has designed CPT codes as part of the national standard for electronic health care transactions:
- Category I: Identify a procedure or service.
- Category II: Identify performance measures, including diagnostic procedures.
- Category III: Identify temporary codes for technology and data collection.

150. A: The ADA provides disabled persons, including those with mental impairment, access to employment and the community. Employers are only allowed to ask applicants if they need accommodations, not if they have disabilities. Applicants may be asked if they can carry out essential functions of a job, not incidental, and medical examinations can only be required after a job is offered. Accommodations can include alterations in a work station, speech recognition software, screen magnifying software, optical character recognition systems, video captioning, Braille readers and screen readers, adapted keyboards and on-screen keyboard, TTYs (text telephones), and amplification systems.

Secret Key #1 - Time is Your Greatest Enemy

Pace Yourself

Wear a watch. At the beginning of the test, check the time (or start a chronometer on your watch to count the minutes), and check the time after every few questions to make sure you are "on schedule."

If you are forced to speed up, do it efficiently. Usually one or more answer choices can be eliminated without too much difficulty. Above all, don't panic. Don't speed up and just begin guessing at random choices. By pacing yourself, and continually monitoring your progress against your watch, you will always know exactly how far ahead or behind you are with your available time. If you find that you are one minute behind on the test, don't skip one question without spending any time on it, just to catch back up. Take 15 fewer seconds on the next four questions, and after four questions you'll have caught back up. Once you catch back up, you can continue working each problem at your normal pace.

Furthermore, don't dwell on the problems that you were rushed on. If a problem was taking up too much time and you made a hurried guess, it must be difficult. The difficult questions are the ones you are most likely to miss anyway, so it isn't a big loss. It is better to end with more time than you need than to run out of time.

Lastly, sometimes it is beneficial to slow down if you are constantly getting ahead of time. You are always more likely to catch a careless mistake by working more slowly than quickly, and among very high-scoring test takers (those who are likely to have lots of time left over), careless errors affect the score more than mastery of material.

Secret Key #2 - Guessing is not Guesswork

You probably know that guessing is a good idea. Unlike other standardized tests, there is no penalty for getting a wrong answer. Even if you have no idea about a question, you still have a 20-25% chance of getting it right.

Most test takers do not understand the impact that proper guessing can have on their score. Unless you score extremely high, guessing will significantly contribute to your final score.

Monkeys Take the Test

What most test takers don't realize is that to insure that 20-25% chance, you have to guess randomly. If you put 20 monkeys in a room to take this test, assuming they answered once per question and behaved themselves, on average they would get 20-25% of the questions correct. Put 20 test takers in the room, and the average will be much lower among guessed questions. Why?
1. The test writers intentionally write deceptive answer choices that "look" right. A test taker has no idea about a question, so he picks the "best looking" answer, which is often wrong. The monkey has no idea what looks good and what doesn't, so it will consistently be right about 20-25% of the time.
2. Test takers will eliminate answer choices from the guessing pool based on a hunch or intuition. Simple but correct answers often get excluded, leaving a 0% chance of being correct. The monkey has no clue, and often gets lucky with the best choice.

This is why the process of elimination endorsed by most test courses is flawed and detrimental to your performance. Test takers don't guess; they make an ignorant stab in the dark that is usually worse than random.

$5 Challenge

Let me introduce one of the most valuable ideas of this course—the $5 challenge:
- *You only mark your "best guess" if you are willing to bet $5 on it.*
- *You only eliminate choices from guessing if you are willing to bet $5 on it.*

Why $5? Five dollars is an amount of money that is small yet not insignificant, and can really add up fast (20 questions could cost you $100). Likewise, each answer choice on one question of the test will have a small impact on your overall score, but it can really add up to a lot of points in the end.

The process of elimination IS valuable. The following shows your chance of guessing it right:

If you eliminate wrong answer choices until only this many remain:	Chance of getting it correct:
1	100%
2	50%
3	33%

However, if you accidentally eliminate the right answer or go on a hunch for an incorrect answer, your chances drop dramatically—to 0%. By guessing among all the answer choices, you are GUARANTEED to have a shot at the right answer.

That's why the $5 test is so valuable. If you give up the advantage and safety of a pure guess, it had better be worth the risk.

What we still haven't covered is how to be sure that whatever guess you make is truly random. Here's the easiest way:
- *Always pick the first answer choice among those remaining.*

Such a technique means that you have decided, **before you see a single test question**, exactly how you are going to guess, and since the order of choices tells you nothing about which one is correct, this guessing technique is perfectly random.

This section is not meant to scare you away from making educated guesses or eliminating choices; you just need to define when a choice is worth eliminating. The $5 test, along with a pre-defined random guessing strategy, is the best way to make sure you reap all of the benefits of guessing.

Secret Key #3 - Practice Smarter, Not Harder

Many test takers delay the test preparation process because they dread the awful amounts of practice time they think necessary to succeed on the test. We have refined an effective method that will take you only a fraction of the time.

There are a number of "obstacles" in the path to success. Among these are answering questions, finishing in time, and mastering test-taking strategies. All must be executed on the day of the test at peak performance, or your score will suffer. The test is a mental marathon that has a large impact on your future.

Just like a marathon runner, it is important to work your way up to the full challenge. So first you just worry about questions, and then time, and finally strategy:

Success Strategy

1. Find a good source for practice tests.
2. If you are willing to make a larger time investment, consider using more than one study guide. Often the different approaches of multiple authors will help you "get" difficult concepts.
3. Take a practice test with no time constraints, with all study helps, "open book." Take your time with questions and focus on applying strategies.
4. Take a practice test with time constraints, with all guides, "open book."
5. Take a final practice test without open material and with time limits.

If you have time to take more practice tests, just repeat step 5. By gradually exposing yourself to the full rigors of the test environment, you will condition your mind to the stress of test day and maximize your success.

Secret Key #4 - Prepare, Don't Procrastinate

Let me state an obvious fact: if you take the test three times, you will probably get three different scores. This is due to the way you feel on test day, the level of preparedness you have, and the version of the test you see. Despite the test writers' claims to the contrary, some versions of the test WILL be easier for you than others.

Since your future depends so much on your score, you should maximize your chances of success. In order to maximize the likelihood of success, you've got to prepare in advance. This means taking practice tests and spending time learning the information and test taking strategies you will need to succeed.

Never go take the actual test as a "practice" test, expecting that you can just take it again if you need to. Take all the practice tests you can on your own, but when you go to take the official test, be prepared, be focused, and do your best the first time!

Secret Key #5 - Test Yourself

Everyone knows that time is money. There is no need to spend too much of your time or too little of your time preparing for the test. You should only spend as much of your precious time preparing as is necessary for you to get the score you need.

Once you have taken a practice test under real conditions of time constraints, then you will know if you are ready for the test or not.

If you have scored extremely high the first time that you take the practice test, then there is not much point in spending countless hours studying. You are already there.

Benchmark your abilities by retaking practice tests and seeing how much you have improved. Once you consistently score high enough to guarantee success, then you are ready.

If you have scored well below where you need, then knuckle down and begin studying in earnest. Check your improvement regularly through the use of practice tests under real conditions. Above all, don't worry, panic, or give up. The key is perseverance!

Then, when you go to take the test, remain confident and remember how well you did on the practice tests. If you can score high enough on a practice test, then you can do the same on the real thing.

General Strategies

The most important thing you can do is to ignore your fears and jump into the test immediately. Do not be overwhelmed by any strange-sounding terms. You have to jump into the test like jumping into a pool—all at once is the easiest way.

Make Predictions

As you read and understand the question, try to guess what the answer will be. Remember that several of the answer choices are wrong, and once you begin reading them, your mind will immediately become cluttered with answer choices designed to throw you off. Your mind is typically the most focused immediately after you have read the question and digested its contents. If you can, try to predict what the correct answer will be. You may be surprised at what you can predict.

Quickly scan the choices and see if your prediction is in the listed answer choices. If it is, then you can be quite confident that you have the right answer. It still won't hurt to check the other answer choices, but most of the time, you've got it!

Answer the Question

It may seem obvious to only pick answer choices that answer the question, but the test writers can create some excellent answer choices that are wrong. Don't pick an answer just because it sounds right, or you believe it to be true. It MUST answer the question. Once you've made your selection, always go back and check it against the question and make sure that you didn't misread the question and that the answer choice does answer the question posed.

Benchmark

After you read the first answer choice, decide if you think it sounds correct or not. If it doesn't, move on to the next answer choice. If it does, mentally mark that answer choice. This doesn't mean that you've definitely selected it as your answer choice, it just means that it's the best you've seen thus far. Go ahead and read the next choice. If the next choice is worse than the one you've already selected, keep going to the next answer choice. If the next choice is better than the choice you've already selected, mentally mark the new answer choice as your best guess.

The first answer choice that you select becomes your standard. Every other answer choice must be benchmarked against that standard. That choice is correct until proven otherwise by another answer choice beating it out. Once you've decided that no other answer choice seems as good, do one final check to ensure that your answer choice answers the question posed.

Valid Information

Don't discount any of the information provided in the question. Every piece of information may be necessary to determine the correct answer. None of the information in the question is there to throw you off (while the answer choices will certainly have information to throw you off). If two seemingly unrelated topics are discussed, don't ignore either. You can be confident there is a relationship, or it wouldn't be included in the question, and you are probably going to have to determine what is that relationship to find the answer.

Avoid "Fact Traps"

Don't get distracted by a choice that is factually true. Your search is for the answer that answers the question. Stay focused and don't fall for an answer that is true but irrelevant. Always go back to the question and make sure you're choosing an answer that actually answers the question and is not just a true statement. An answer can be factually correct, but it MUST answer the question asked. Additionally, two answers can both be seemingly correct, so be sure to read all of the answer choices, and make sure that you get the one that BEST answers the question.

Milk the Question

Some of the questions may throw you completely off. They might deal with a subject you have not been exposed to, or one that you haven't reviewed in years. While your lack of knowledge about the subject will be a hindrance, the question itself can give you many clues that will help you find the correct answer. Read the question carefully and look for clues. Watch particularly for adjectives and nouns describing difficult terms or words that you don't recognize. Regardless of whether you completely understand a word or not, replacing it with a synonym, either provided or one you more familiar with, may help you to understand what the questions are asking. Rather than wracking your mind about specific detailed information concerning a difficult term or word, try to use mental substitutes that are easier to understand.

The Trap of Familiarity

Don't just choose a word because you recognize it. On difficult questions, you may not recognize a number of words in the answer choices. The test writers don't put "make-believe" words on the test, so don't think that just because you only recognize all the words in one answer choice that that answer choice must be correct. If you only recognize words in one answer choice, then focus on that one. Is it correct? Try your best to determine if it is correct. If it is, that's great. If not, eliminate it. Each word and answer choice you eliminate increases your chances of getting the question correct, even if you then have to guess among the unfamiliar choices.

Eliminate Answers

Eliminate choices as soon as you realize they are wrong. But be careful! Make sure you consider all of the possible answer choices. Just because one appears right, doesn't mean that the next one won't be even better! The test writers will usually put more than one good answer choice for every question, so read all of them. Don't worry if you are stuck between two that seem right. By getting down to just two remaining possible choices, your odds are now 50/50. Rather than wasting too much time, play the odds. You are guessing, but guessing wisely because you've been able to knock out some of the answer choices that you know are wrong. If you are eliminating choices and realize that the last answer choice you are left with is also obviously wrong, don't panic. Start over and consider each choice again. There may easily be something that you missed the first time and will realize on the second pass.

Tough Questions

If you are stumped on a problem or it appears too hard or too difficult, don't waste time. Move on! Remember though, if you can quickly check for obviously incorrect answer choices, your chances of guessing correctly are greatly improved. Before you completely give up, at least try to knock out a couple of possible answers. Eliminate what you can and then guess at the remaining answer choices before moving on.

Brainstorm

If you get stuck on a difficult question, spend a few seconds quickly brainstorming. Run through the complete list of possible answer choices. Look at each choice and ask yourself, "Could this answer the question satisfactorily?" Go through each answer choice and consider it independently of the others. By systematically going through all possibilities, you may find something that you would otherwise overlook. Remember though that when you get stuck, it's important to try to keep moving.

Read Carefully

Understand the problem. Read the question and answer choices carefully. Don't miss the question because you misread the terms. You have plenty of time to read each question thoroughly and make sure you understand what is being asked. Yet a happy medium must be attained, so don't waste too much time. You must read carefully, but efficiently.

Face Value

When in doubt, use common sense. Always accept the situation in the problem at face value. Don't read too much into it. These problems will not require you to make huge leaps of logic. The test writers aren't trying to throw you off with a cheap trick. If you have to go beyond creativity and make a leap of logic in order to have an answer choice answer the question, then you should look at the other answer choices. Don't overcomplicate the problem by creating theoretical relationships or explanations that will warp time or space. These are normal problems rooted in reality. It's just that the applicable relationship or explanation may not be readily apparent and you have to figure things out. Use your common sense to interpret anything that isn't clear.

Prefixes

If you're having trouble with a word in the question or answer choices, try dissecting it. Take advantage of every clue that the word might include. Prefixes and suffixes can be a huge help. Usually they allow you to determine a basic meaning. Pre- means before, post- means after, pro - is positive, de- is negative. From these prefixes and suffixes, you can get an idea of the general meaning of the word and try to put it into context. Beware though of any traps. Just because con- is the opposite of pro-, doesn't necessarily mean congress is the opposite of progress!

Hedge Phrases

Watch out for critical hedge phrases, led off with words such as "likely," "may," "can," "sometimes," "often," "almost," "mostly," "usually," "generally," "rarely," and "sometimes." Question writers insert these hedge phrases to cover every possibility. Often an answer choice will be wrong simply because it leaves no room for exception. Unless the situation calls for them, avoid answer choices that have definitive words like "exactly," and "always."

Switchback Words

Stay alert for "switchbacks." These are the words and phrases frequently used to alert you to shifts in thought. The most common switchback word is "but." Others include "although," "however," "nevertheless," "on the other hand," "even though," "while," "in spite of," "despite," and "regardless of."

New Information

Correct answer choices will rarely have completely new information included. Answer choices typically are straightforward reflections of the material asked about and will directly relate to the question. If a new piece of information is included in an answer choice that doesn't even seem to relate to the topic being asked about, then that answer choice is likely incorrect. All of the information needed to answer the question is usually provided for you in the question. You should not have to make guesses that are unsupported or choose answer choices that require unknown information that cannot be reasoned from what is given.

Time Management

On technical questions, don't get lost on the technical terms. Don't spend too much time on any one question. If you don't know what a term means, then odds are you aren't going to get much further since you don't have a dictionary. You should be able to immediately recognize whether or not you know a term. If you don't, work with the other clues that you have—the other answer choices and terms provided—but don't waste too much time trying to figure out a difficult term that you don't know.

Contextual Clues

Look for contextual clues. An answer can be right but not the correct answer. The contextual clues will help you find the answer that is most right and is correct. Understand the context in which a phrase or statement is made. This will help you make important distinctions.

Don't Panic

Panicking will not answer any questions for you; therefore, it isn't helpful. When you first see the question, if your mind goes blank, take a deep breath. Force yourself to mechanically go through the steps of solving the problem using the strategies you've learned.

Pace Yourself

Don't get clock fever. It's easy to be overwhelmed when you're looking at a page full of questions, your mind is full of random thoughts and feeling confused, and the clock is ticking down faster than you would like. Calm down and maintain the pace that you have set for yourself. As long as you are on track by monitoring your pace, you are guaranteed to have enough time for yourself. When you get to the last few minutes of the test, it may seem like you won't have enough time left, but if you only have as many questions as you should have left at that point, then you're right on track!

Answer Selection

The best way to pick an answer choice is to eliminate all of those that are wrong, until only one is left and confirm that is the correct answer. Sometimes though, an answer choice may immediately look right. Be careful! Take a second to make sure that the other choices are not equally obvious. Don't make a hasty mistake. There are only two times that you should stop before checking other answers. First is when you are positive that the answer choice you have selected is correct. Second is when time is almost out and you have to make a quick guess!

Check Your Work

Since you will probably not know every term listed and the answer to every question, it is important that you get credit for the ones that you do know. Don't miss any questions through careless mistakes. If at all possible, try to take a second to look back over your answer selection and make sure you've selected the correct answer choice and haven't made a costly careless mistake (such as marking an answer choice that you didn't mean to mark). The time it takes for this quick double check should more than pay for itself in caught mistakes.

Beware of Directly Quoted Answers

Sometimes an answer choice will repeat word for word a portion of the question or reference section. However, beware of such exact duplication. It may be a trap! More than likely, the correct choice will paraphrase or summarize a point, rather than being exactly the same wording.

Slang

Scientific sounding answers are better than slang ones. An answer choice that begins "To compare the outcomes…" is much more likely to be correct than one that begins "Because some people insisted…"

Extreme Statements

Avoid wild answers that throw out highly controversial ideas that are proclaimed as established fact. An answer choice that states the "process should used in certain situations, if…" is much more likely to be correct than one that states the "process should be discontinued completely." The first is a calm rational statement and doesn't even make a definitive, uncompromising stance, using a hedge word "if" to provide wiggle room, whereas the second choice is a radical idea and far more extreme.

Answer Choice Families

When you have two or more answer choices that are direct opposites or parallels, one of them is usually the correct answer. For instance, if one answer choice states "x increases" and another answer choice states "x decreases" or "y increases," then those two or three answer choices are very similar in construction and fall into the same family of answer choices. A family of answer choices consists of two or three answer choices, very similar in construction, but often with directly opposite meanings. Usually the correct answer choice will be in that family of answer choices. The "odd man out" or answer choice that doesn't seem to fit the parallel construction of the other answer choices is more likely to be incorrect.

Special Report: How to Overcome Test Anxiety

The very nature of tests caters to some level of anxiety, nervousness, or tension, just as we feel for any important event that occurs in our lives. A little bit of anxiety or nervousness can be a good thing. It helps us with motivation, and makes achievement just that much sweeter. However, too much anxiety can be a problem, especially if it hinders our ability to function and perform.

"Test anxiety," is the term that refers to the emotional reactions that some test-takers experience when faced with a test or exam. Having a fear of testing and exams is based upon a rational fear, since the test-taker's performance can shape the course of an academic career. Nevertheless, experiencing excessive fear of examinations will only interfere with the test-taker's ability to perform and chance to be successful.

There are a large variety of causes that can contribute to the development and sensation of test anxiety. These include, but are not limited to, lack of preparation and worrying about issues surrounding the test.

Lack of Preparation

Lack of preparation can be identified by the following behaviors or situations:
- Not scheduling enough time to study, and therefore cramming the night before the test or exam
- Managing time poorly, to create the sensation that there is not enough time to do everything
- Failing to organize the text information in advance, so that the study material consists of the entire text and not simply the pertinent information
- Poor overall studying habits

Worrying, on the other hand, can be related to both the test taker, or many other factors around him/her that will be affected by the results of the test. These include worrying about:
- Previous performances on similar exams, or exams in general
- How friends and other students are achieving
- The negative consequences that will result from a poor grade or failure

There are three primary elements to test anxiety. Physical components, which involve the same typical bodily reactions as those to acute anxiety (to be discussed below). Emotional factors have to do with fear or panic. Mental or cognitive issues concerning attention spans and memory abilities.

Physical Signals

There are many different symptoms of test anxiety, and these are not limited to mental and emotional strain. Frequently there are a range of physical signals that will let a test taker know that he/she is suffering from test anxiety. These bodily changes can include the following:

- Perspiring
- Sweaty palms
- Wet, trembling hands
- Nausea
- Dry mouth
- A knot in the stomach
- Headache
- Faintness
- Muscle tension
- Aching shoulders, back and neck
- Rapid heart beat
- Feeling too hot/cold

To recognize the sensation of test anxiety, a test-taker should monitor him/herself for the following sensations:

- The physical distress symptoms as listed above
- Emotional sensitivity, expressing emotional feelings such as the need to cry or laugh too much, or a sensation of anger or helplessness
- A decreased ability to think, causing the test-taker to blank out or have racing thoughts that are hard to organize or control.

Though most students will feel some level of anxiety when faced with a test or exam, the majority can cope with that anxiety and maintain it at a manageable level. However, those who cannot are faced with a very real and very serious condition, which can and should be controlled for the immeasurable benefit of this sufferer.

Naturally, these sensations lead to negative results for the testing experience. The most common effects of test anxiety have to do with nervousness and mental blocking.

Nervousness

Nervousness can appear in several different levels:

- The test-taker's difficulty, or even inability to read and understand the questions on the test
- The difficulty or inability to organize thoughts to a coherent form
- The difficulty or inability to recall key words and concepts relating to the testing questions (especially essays)
- The receipt of poor grades on a test, though the test material was well known by the test taker

Conversely, a person may also experience mental blocking, which involves:

- Blanking out on test questions
- Only remembering the correct answers to the questions when the test has already finished.

Fortunately for test anxiety sufferers, beating these feelings, to a large degree, has to do with proper preparation. When a test taker has a feeling of preparedness, then anxiety will be dramatically lessened.

The first step to resolving anxiety issues is to distinguish which of the two types of anxiety are being suffered. If the anxiety is a direct result of a lack of preparation, this should be considered a normal reaction, and the anxiety level (as opposed to the test results) shouldn't be anything to worry about. However, if, when adequately prepared, the test-taker still panics, blanks out, or seems to overreact, this is not a fully rational reaction. While this can be considered normal too, there are many ways to combat and overcome these effects.

Remember that anxiety cannot be entirely eliminated, however, there are ways to minimize it, to make the anxiety easier to manage. Preparation is one of the best ways to minimize test anxiety. Therefore the following techniques are wise in order to best fight off any anxiety that may want to build.

To begin with, try to avoid cramming before a test, whenever it is possible. By trying to memorize an entire term's worth of information in one day, you'll be shocking your system, and not giving yourself a very good chance to absorb the information. This is an easy path to anxiety, so for those who suffer from test anxiety, cramming should not even be considered an option.

Instead of cramming, work throughout the semester to combine all of the material which is presented throughout the semester, and work on it gradually as the course goes by, making sure to master the main concepts first, leaving minor details for a week or so before the test.

To study for the upcoming exam, be sure to pose questions that may be on the examination, to gauge the ability to answer them by integrating the ideas from your texts, notes and lectures, as well as any supplementary readings.

If it is truly impossible to cover all of the information that was covered in that particular term, concentrate on the most important portions, that can be covered very well. Learn these concepts as best as possible, so that when the test comes, a goal can be made to use these concepts as presentations of your knowledge.

In addition to study habits, changes in attitude are critical to beating a struggle with test anxiety. In fact, an improvement of the perspective over the entire test-taking experience can actually help a test taker to enjoy studying and therefore improve the overall experience. Be certain not to overemphasize the significance of the grade - know that the result of the test is neither a reflection of self worth, nor is it a measure of intelligence; one grade will not predict a person's future success.

To improve an overall testing outlook, the following steps should be tried:
- Keeping in mind that the most reasonable expectation for taking a test is to expect to try to demonstrate as much of what you know as you possibly can.
- Reminding ourselves that a test is only one test; this is not the only one, and there will be others.
- The thought of thinking of oneself in an irrational, all-or-nothing term should be avoided at all costs.

A reward should be designated for after the test, so there's something to look forward to. Whether it be going to a movie, going out to eat, or simply visiting friends, schedule it in advance, and do it no matter what result is expected on the exam.

Test-takers should also keep in mind that the basics are some of the most important things, even beyond anti-anxiety techniques and studying. Never neglect the basic social, emotional and biological needs, in order to try to absorb information. In order to best achieve, these three factors must be held as just as important as the studying itself.

Study Steps

Remember the following important steps for studying:
- Maintain healthy nutrition and exercise habits. Continue both your recreational activities and social pass times. These both contribute to your physical and emotional well being.
- Be certain to get a good amount of sleep, especially the night before the test, because when you're overtired you are not able to perform to the best of your best ability.
- Keep the studying pace to a moderate level by taking breaks when they are needed, and varying the work whenever possible, to keep the mind fresh instead of getting bored.
- When enough studying has been done that all the material that can be learned has been learned, and the test taker is prepared for the test, stop studying and do something relaxing such as listening to music, watching a movie, or taking a warm bubble bath.

There are also many other techniques to minimize the uneasiness or apprehension that is experienced along with test anxiety before, during, or even after the examination. In fact, there are a great deal of things that can be done to stop anxiety from interfering with lifestyle and performance. Again, remember that anxiety will not be eliminated entirely, and it shouldn't be. Otherwise that "up" feeling for exams would not exist, and most of us depend on that sensation to perform better than usual. However, this anxiety has to be at a level that is manageable.

Of course, as we have just discussed, being prepared for the exam is half the battle right away. Attending all classes, finding out what knowledge will be expected on the exam, and knowing the exam schedules are easy steps to lowering anxiety. Keeping up with work will remove the need to cram, and efficient study habits will eliminate wasted time. Studying should be done in an ideal location for concentration, so that it is simple to become interested in the material and give it complete attention. A method such as SQ3R (Survey, Question, Read, Recite, Review) is a wonderful key to follow to make sure that the study habits are as effective as possible, especially in the case of learning from a textbook. Flashcards are great techniques for memorization. Learning to take good notes will mean that notes will be full of useful information, so that less sifting will need to be done to seek out what is pertinent for studying. Reviewing notes after class and then again on occasion will keep the information fresh in the mind. From notes that have been taken summary sheets and outlines can be made for simpler reviewing.

A study group can also be a very motivational and helpful place to study, as there will be a sharing of ideas, all of the minds can work together, to make sure that everyone understands, and the studying will be made more interesting because it will be a social occasion.

Basically, though, as long as the test-taker remains organized and self confident, with efficient study habits, less time will need to be spent studying, and higher grades will be achieved.

To become self confident, there are many useful steps. The first of these is "self talk." It has been shown through extensive research, that self-talk for students who suffer from test anxiety, should be well monitored, in order to make sure that it contributes to self confidence as opposed to sinking the student. Frequently the self talk of test-anxious students is negative or self-defeating, thinking that everyone else is smarter and faster, that they always mess up, and that if they don't do well, they'll fail the entire course. It is important to decreasing anxiety that awareness is made of self talk. Try writing any negative self thoughts and then disputing them with a positive statement instead. Begin self-encouragement as though it was a friend speaking. Repeat positive statements to help reprogram the mind to believing in successes instead of failures.

Helpful Techniques

Other extremely helpful techniques include:
- Self-visualization of doing well and reaching goals
- While aiming for an "A" level of understanding, don't try to "overprotect" by setting your expectations lower. This will only convince the mind to stop studying in order to meet the lower expectations.
- Don't make comparisons with the results or habits of other students. These are individual factors, and different things work for different people, causing different results.
- Strive to become an expert in learning what works well, and what can be done in order to improve. Consider collecting this data in a journal.
- Create rewards for after studying instead of doing things before studying that will only turn into avoidance behaviors.
- Make a practice of relaxing - by using methods such as progressive relaxation, self-hypnosis, guided imagery, etc - in order to make relaxation an automatic sensation.
- Work on creating a state of relaxed concentration so that concentrating will take on the focus of the mind, so that none will be wasted on worrying.
- Take good care of the physical self by eating well and getting enough sleep.
- Plan in time for exercise and stick to this plan.

Beyond these techniques, there are other methods to be used before, during and after the test that will help the test-taker perform well in addition to overcoming anxiety.

Before the exam comes the academic preparation. This involves establishing a study schedule and beginning at least one week before the actual date of the test. By doing this, the anxiety of not having enough time to study for the test will be automatically eliminated. Moreover, this will make the studying a much more effective experience, ensuring that the learning will be an easier process. This relieves much undue pressure on the test-taker.

Summary sheets, note cards, and flash cards with the main concepts and examples of these main concepts should be prepared in advance of the actual studying time. A topic should never be eliminated from this process. By omitting a topic because it isn't expected to be on the test is only setting up the test-taker for anxiety should it actually appear on the exam. Utilize the course syllabus for laying out the topics that should be studied. Carefully go over the notes that were made in class, paying special attention to any of the issues that the professor took special care to emphasize while lecturing in class. In the textbooks, use the chapter review, or if possible, the chapter tests, to begin your review.

It may even be possible to ask the instructor what information will be covered on the exam, or what the format of the exam will be (for example, multiple choice, essay, free form, true-false). Additionally, see if it is possible to find out how many questions will be on the test. If a review sheet or sample test has been offered by the professor, make good use of it, above anything else, for the preparation for the test. Another great resource for getting to know the examination is reviewing tests from previous semesters. Use these tests to review, and aim to achieve a 100% score on each of the possible topics. With a few exceptions, the goal that you set for yourself is the highest one that you will reach.

Take all of the questions that were assigned as homework, and rework them to any other possible course material. The more problems reworked, the more skill and confidence will form as a result. When forming the solution to a problem, write out each of the steps. Don't simply do head work. By doing as many steps on paper as possible, much clarification and therefore confidence will be formed. Do this with as many homework problems as possible, before checking the answers. By checking the answer after each problem, a reinforcement will exist, that will not be on the exam. Study situations should be as exam-like as possible, to prime the test-taker's system for the experience. By waiting to check the answers at the end, a psychological advantage will be formed, to decrease the stress factor.

Another fantastic reason for not cramming is the avoidance of confusion in concepts, especially when it comes to mathematics. 8-10 hours of study will become one hundred percent more effective if it is spread out over a week or at least several days, instead of doing it all in one sitting. Recognize that the human brain requires time in order to assimilate new material, so frequent breaks and a span of study time over several days will be much more beneficial.

Additionally, don't study right up until the point of the exam. Studying should stop a minimum of one hour before the exam begins. This allows the brain to rest and put things in their proper order. This will also provide the time to become as relaxed as possible when going into the examination room. The test-taker will also have time to eat well and eat sensibly. Know that the brain needs food as much as the rest of the body. With enough food and enough sleep, as well as a relaxed attitude, the body and the mind are primed for success.

Avoid any anxious classmates who are talking about the exam. These students only spread anxiety, and are not worth sharing the anxious sentimentalities.

Before the test also involves creating a positive attitude, so mental preparation should also be a point of concentration. There are many keys to creating a positive attitude. Should fears become rushing in, make a visualization of taking the exam, doing well, and seeing an A written on the paper. Write out a list of affirmations that will bring a feeling of confidence, such as "I am doing well in my English class," "I studied well and know my material," "I enjoy this class." Even if the affirmations aren't believed at first, it sends a positive message to the subconscious which will result in an alteration of the overall belief system, which is the system that creates reality.

If a sensation of panic begins, work with the fear and imagine the very worst! Work through the entire scenario of not passing the test, failing the entire course, and dropping out of school, followed by not getting a job, and pushing a shopping cart through the dark alley where you'll live. This will place things into perspective! Then, practice deep breathing and create a visualization of the opposite situation - achieving an "A" on the exam, passing the entire course, receiving the degree at a graduation ceremony.

On the day of the test, there are many things to be done to ensure the best results, as well as the most calm outlook. The following stages are suggested in order to maximize test-taking potential:

- Begin the examination day with a moderate breakfast, and avoid any coffee or beverages with caffeine if the test taker is prone to jitters. Even people who are used to managing caffeine can feel jittery or light-headed when it is taken on a test day.
- Attempt to do something that is relaxing before the examination begins. As last minute cramming clouds the mastering of overall concepts, it is better to use this time to create a calming outlook.
- Be certain to arrive at the test location well in advance, in order to provide time to select a location that is away from doors, windows and other distractions, as well as giving enough time to relax before the test begins.
- Keep away from anxiety generating classmates who will upset the sensation of stability and relaxation that is being attempted before the exam.
- Should the waiting period before the exam begins cause anxiety, create a self-distraction by reading a light magazine or something else that is relaxing and simple.

During the exam itself, read the entire exam from beginning to end, and find out how much time should be allotted to each individual problem. Once writing the exam, should more time be taken for a problem, it should be abandoned, in order to begin another problem. If there is time at the end, the unfinished problem can always be returned to and completed.

Read the instructions very carefully - twice - so that unpleasant surprises won't follow during or after the exam has ended.

When writing the exam, pretend that the situation is actually simply the completion of homework within a library, or at home. This will assist in forming a relaxed atmosphere, and will allow the brain extra focus for the complex thinking function.

Begin the exam with all of the questions with which the most confidence is felt. This will build the confidence level regarding the entire exam and will begin a quality momentum. This will also create encouragement for trying the problems where uncertainty resides.

Going with the "gut instinct" is always the way to go when solving a problem. Second guessing should be avoided at all costs. Have confidence in the ability to do well.

For essay questions, create an outline in advance that will keep the mind organized and make certain that all of the points are remembered. For multiple choice, read every answer, even if the correct one has been spotted - a better one may exist.

Continue at a pace that is reasonable and not rushed, in order to be able to work carefully. Provide enough time to go over the answers at the end, to check for small errors that can be corrected.

Should a feeling of panic begin, breathe deeply, and think of the feeling of the body releasing sand through its pores. Visualize a calm, peaceful place, and include all of the sights, sounds and sensations of this image. Continue the deep breathing, and take a few minutes to continue this with closed eyes. When all is well again, return to the test.

If a "blanking" occurs for a certain question, skip it and move on to the next question. There will be time to return to the other question later. Get everything done that can be done, first, to guarantee all the grades that can be compiled, and to build all of the confidence possible. Then return to the weaker questions to build the marks from there.

Remember, one's own reality can be created, so as long as the belief is there, success will follow. And remember: anxiety can happen later, right now, there's an exam to be written!

After the examination is complete, whether there is a feeling for a good grade or a bad grade, don't dwell on the exam, and be certain to follow through on the reward that was promised...and enjoy it! Don't dwell on any mistakes that have been made, as there is nothing that can be done at this point anyway.

Additionally, don't begin to study for the next test right away. Do something relaxing for a while, and let the mind relax and prepare itself to begin absorbing information again.

From the results of the exam - both the grade and the entire experience, be certain to learn from what has gone on. Perfect studying habits and work some more on confidence in order to make the next examination experience even better than the last one.

Learn to avoid places where openings occurred for laziness, procrastination and day dreaming.

Use the time between this exam and the next one to better learn to relax, even learning to relax on cue, so that any anxiety can be controlled during the next exam. Learn how to relax the body. Slouch in your chair if that helps. Tighten and then relax all of the different muscle groups, one group at a time, beginning with the feet and then working all the way up to the neck and face. This will ultimately relax the muscles more than they were to begin with. Learn how to breathe deeply and comfortably, and focus on this breathing going in and out as a relaxing thought. With every exhale, repeat the word "relax."

As common as test anxiety is, it is very possible to overcome it. Make yourself one of the test-takers who overcome this frustrating hindrance.

Additional Bonus Material

Due to our efforts to try to keep this book to a manageable length, we've created a link that will give you access to all of your additional bonus material.

Please visit http://www.mometrix.com/bonus948/infonurse to access the information.